Three Minds, One Brain

A Practical Guide to Untangling and Treating
Quiet BPD, ADHD, and Autism Overlap

The Research Is Clear:

Approximately 30-60% of people with BPD also have ADHD.
Between 50-70% of autistic people meet ADHD criteria. BPD
features appear in high-masking autistic populations at significant
rates. When these conditions overlap, outcomes improve dramatically
with integrated treatment—but only when properly recognized.

Katie June Rangel

Three Minds, One Brain: A Practical Guide to Untangling and Treating Quiet BPD, ADHD, and Autism Overlap

ISBN: 978-1-923604-75-9

First Edition: 2025

This book is designed to provide information and guidance regarding the overlap between Quiet Borderline Personality Disorder, ADHD, and Autism Spectrum Disorder. It is sold with the understanding that the publisher and author are not engaged in rendering psychological, medical, or other professional services. If expert assistance or counseling is needed, the services of a competent professional should be sought.

The purpose of this book is to educate and inform. The author and publisher shall have neither liability nor responsibility to any person or entity with respect to any loss or damage caused, or alleged to have been caused, directly or indirectly, by the information contained in this book.

Every effort has been made to ensure the accuracy of the information presented. However, mental health is a rapidly evolving field, and new research may modify or contradict information presented here. Readers should consult current research and qualified professionals when making treatment decisions.

The case examples, scenarios, and personal stories presented in this book are composites drawn from multiple sources, clinical literature, research studies, and the author's professional experience. All names, identifying details, and specific circumstances have been changed or fictionalized to protect privacy. Any resemblance to actual persons, living or deceased, or actual events is purely coincidental.

The names Maria, Jake, Emma, Alex, Sarah, Marcus, Taylor, Jordan, David, Rachel, Sophie, Olivia, Lucas, Maya, Ethan, Ava, Isabella, Noah, and all other names used throughout this text are pseudonyms created solely for illustrative and educational purposes. These names do not refer to any actual individuals, clients, or patients.

References to diagnostic criteria, assessment tools, and therapeutic approaches (including but not limited to DSM-5-TR criteria, DBT skills, trauma-informed approaches, and neurodiversity frameworks) are provided for educational purposes. Implementation of any assessment or treatment approach requires appropriate professional training, supervision, and licensure.

Table of Contents

Chapter 1: When Nothing Quite Fits

Understanding the Quiet Presentations

You've probably spent years wondering why you feel so different from everyone else, yet no single diagnosis ever quite captures your experience. Maybe you've collected diagnoses like puzzle pieces that don't quite fit together, or perhaps you're still searching for answers while therapists keep changing their minds about what's "wrong" with you.

Here's what might surprise you: if you're struggling to find a diagnosis that fits, it's not because you're difficult or making things up. You might be experiencing what happens when ADHD, autism, and borderline personality disorder overlap or hide behind each other – especially in their "quiet" forms that often go unrecognized for decades.

The Hidden Epidemic of Quiet Presentations

When we think of ADHD, we might picture a hyperactive child bouncing off walls. When we imagine autism, we might envision someone who can't make eye contact or speak. And when we consider borderline personality disorder, we might think of dramatic outbursts and hospital visits. But what if I told you that all three conditions can present so quietly that even experienced clinicians miss them?

The quiet presentations look different. In quiet ADHD, the chaos happens entirely inside your head – a thousand browser tabs open in your mind while you appear calm on the surface. In autism, you might have learned to force eye contact until it hurts, rehearse conversations in advance, and hide your sensory overwhelm behind a carefully constructed mask. In quiet BPD, instead of explosive anger, you turn everything inward – the rage becomes self-hatred, the fear of abandonment becomes people-pleasing, and the identity confusion becomes shape-shifting to match whoever you're with.

These quiet presentations share something crucial: they're exhausting. You're working overtime just to appear "normal," and nobody sees the tremendous effort it takes. Research shows that 80% of autistic women are initially misdiagnosed, often with conditions like BPD, anxiety, or depression. Why? Because the diagnostic criteria were built around how these conditions look in young boys and men, not how they manifest in women, non-binary individuals, or anyone who's learned to hide their struggles.

When Conditions Collide: The Overlap Nobody Talks About

Here's a statistic that might validate everything you've been experiencing: 33.7% of people with ADHD also meet criteria for BPD, compared to just 5.2% of the general population. That's not a coincidence – it's a massive overlap that most professionals aren't trained to recognize.

Think about it this way: ADHD affects your ability to regulate attention and impulses. Autism affects how you process sensory information and social cues. BPD affects your sense of self and emotional regulation. Now imagine having all three, or traits of all three, operating simultaneously. No wonder you feel like you're fighting multiple battles at once.

The overlap creates a perfect storm of confusion. Your ADHD impulsivity might look like BPD self-destructive behavior. Your autistic need for routine might be mistaken for BPD's frantic efforts to avoid abandonment (because change feels like abandonment to your nervous system). Your BPD identity confusion might actually be autistic masking – you've been copying others for so long that you don't know who you really are.

The Masking Phenomenon: Your Invisible Superpower and Your Greatest Burden

Masking is what happens when you consciously or unconsciously hide your neurodivergent traits to fit in. It's the script you run in social situations, the energy you spend monitoring your body language, the exhaustion that hits after a "normal" day at work. Research on autistic masking shows it's associated with increased anxiety, depression, and suicidal ideation – because pretending to be someone you're not is literally killing you.

But here's where it gets complicated: each condition involves its own type of masking. ADHD masking might mean sitting still in meetings while your mind races, creating elaborate systems to remember things everyone else seems to track effortlessly, or overcompensating for time blindness by arriving everywhere an hour early. Autism masking involves copying others' social behaviors, suppressing stims, and ignoring sensory discomfort until you collapse. BPD masking means hiding your emotional storms, pretending you have a stable sense of self, and managing fear of abandonment by never showing need.

When you're masking multiple conditions simultaneously, the cognitive load becomes overwhelming. You're not just hiding one aspect of yourself – you're managing multiple hidden selves, each with different needs and expressions. No wonder you're exhausted. No wonder you sometimes don't know who you really are.

The Cost of Being Misunderstood

What happens when these overlapping conditions go unrecognized? You get labeled as "difficult," "treatment-resistant," or "attention-seeking." You might spend years in therapy that doesn't help because it's targeting the wrong condition. You might be medicated for depression when you're actually experiencing autistic burnout, or treated for anxiety when you're dealing with ADHD restlessness.

The mental health costs are staggering. People with undiagnosed or misdiagnosed neurodevelopmental conditions have higher rates of anxiety, depression, eating disorders, and substance abuse. Why? Because when you don't understand your brain, you can't work with

3

it. You end up fighting against yourself, trying to force your square-peg brain into round holes, and blaming yourself when it doesn't work.

But there's another cost that's harder to measure: the loss of self. When you've spent decades not knowing why you're different, you internalize the message that something is fundamentally wrong with you. You might have heard "you're too sensitive," "you're overreacting," "you just need to try harder," or "you're making excuses" so many times that these became your internal soundtrack.

Recognizing Yourself in the Patterns

Let's get specific about what these quiet, overlapping presentations actually look like in daily life. You might recognize yourself in these patterns:

You have what feels like emotional whiplash – intense feelings that seem to come from nowhere, but when you look closer, they're triggered by sensory overwhelm (autism), rejection sensitivity (ADHD), or fear of abandonment (BPD). Sometimes it's all three at once, and you can't untangle which is which.

Your relationships are complicated. You desperately want connection but find people exhausting. You might cycle between intense attachment and needing complete solitude. You mirror others so well that different people know completely different versions of you, and you're not sure which one is real.

Your executive function is inconsistent. Some days you can hyperfocus for hours; other days, you can't start the simplest task. This isn't laziness – it's the intersection of ADHD executive dysfunction, autistic inertia, and BPD emotional dysregulation affecting your ability to function.

You have sensory issues that seem to fluctuate. Sometimes you don't notice sensory input at all (ADHD hyposensitivity); sometimes it's overwhelming (autistic sensory processing differences); sometimes

4

your emotional state determines your sensory tolerance (BPD emotional dysregulation affecting sensory processing).

Your sense of self feels unstable, but you're not sure if it's BPD identity disturbance, autistic masking, or ADHD inconsistency. Maybe it's all three, layered on top of each other like geological strata, each one affecting how the others manifest.

Breaking Free from the Diagnostic Box

Here's something revolutionary to consider: maybe you don't fit neatly into one diagnostic box because human brains don't actually work in neat categories. The DSM and ICD are attempts to organize the beautiful chaos of human neurodiversity into discrete units, but real brains are messier than that.

Research is beginning to catch up to what many of us have known all along – these conditions share genetic factors, brain differences, and lived experiences. They're not completely separate entities but overlapping circles in a complex Venn diagram. Understanding this overlap isn't just academic; it's the key to finally making sense of your experience.

This understanding changes everything. Instead of seeing yourself as "failing" at having ADHD because you also have autistic traits, or being "bad at" BPD because your emotional dysregulation looks different, you can recognize that you're navigating multiple neurological differences that interact in complex ways.

Your Journey Forward Starts Here

Reading this chapter might feel like looking in a mirror for the first time – seeing yourself reflected accurately after years of distorted images. That recognition might bring relief, grief, anger, or all of the above. These feelings are valid. You've likely spent years being misunderstood, pathologized, or dismissed. Discovering that your struggles have a name – or multiple names – and that you're not alone in experiencing them can be overwhelming.

But here's what I want you to know: understanding your brain's unique wiring isn't about collecting labels or diagnoses. It's about finally having a map for the territory you've been navigating blind. It's about replacing self-blame with self-understanding, confusion with clarity, and isolation with community.

The journey ahead won't always be easy. Untangling these overlapping conditions takes time, patience, and often professional support. But you've already done the hardest part – you've survived this long without a proper map. Now, we're going to build one together.

Self-Assessment Checklist: Signs You Might Have Been Misdiagnosed

Consider whether these experiences resonate with you:

- Your diagnosis seems to explain some symptoms but not others

- Treatments that work for others with your diagnosis don't work for you

- You've received multiple different diagnoses over the years

- Professionals seem confused by your presentation

- You relate more to online communities than clinical descriptions

- Your symptoms seem to change depending on stress, environment, or life circumstances

- You've been called "treatment-resistant" or "complicated"

- Standard therapy approaches feel incomplete or wrong

- You mask so well that professionals don't believe your struggles

- Your internal experience doesn't match what others observe

Timeline Worksheet: Mapping Your Diagnostic Journey

Take some time to map out your journey:

1. When did you first notice you were different?

2. What was your first contact with mental health services?

3. What diagnoses have you received, and when?

4. Which treatments have you tried, and how did they work?

5. When did you start questioning your diagnosis?

6. What led you to explore these overlapping conditions?

This timeline isn't about getting it perfect – it's about seeing patterns in your journey and recognizing how your understanding of yourself has evolved.

Now that you've explored this territory of quiet presentations and overlapping conditions, you're ready to dive deeper into why these conditions get confused in the first place. The diagnostic maze awaits, but you're no longer walking through it alone.

Chapter 2: The Diagnostic Maze

Why These Conditions Get Confused

You sit across from yet another mental health professional, trying to explain your inner world in the ten minutes they've allotted for "history taking." They nod, type notes, and then confidently declare you have anxiety and depression. But something feels off – like they've seen your shadow on the wall and mistaken it for your whole being.

This scenario plays out thousands of times daily in clinics worldwide. Well-meaning professionals, armed with diagnostic manuals designed decades ago, try to fit complex human experiences into rigid categories. When you present with overlapping traits of ADHD, autism, and BPD – especially in their quieter forms – the diagnostic process becomes a maze where even experienced clinicians can get lost.

The Evolution of Understanding: How We Got Here

The diagnostic criteria we use today weren't handed down from some all-knowing authority – they evolved through decades of observation, mostly of white male children in clinical settings. The DSM-5, published in 2013, made some progress in recognizing autism in females and adults, but the criteria still lean heavily toward external, observable behaviors rather than internal experiences.

The recent DSM-5-TR update in 2022 finally acknowledged that autism symptoms "may be masked by learned strategies in later life." This single sentence represents a revolution in thinking – an admission that people can be autistic without fitting the stereotypical presentation. Similarly, the ICD-11 has begun recognizing that

ADHD and autism can co-occur, overturning decades of diagnostic rules that said you couldn't have both.

But here's the problem: most practicing clinicians trained before these updates. They learned that autism and ADHD were childhood conditions, primarily affecting boys. They learned that BPD was a "difficult" diagnosis, often applied to women with trauma histories. They didn't learn about masking, camouflaging, or how these conditions manifest differently across genders and cultures.

This historical context matters because it explains why you might have been misdiagnosed. It's not that previous clinicians were incompetent – they were working with outdated maps, trying to navigate new territory with old tools.

The Gender Bias Built Into Diagnosis

Let's be honest about something uncomfortable: the entire diagnostic system was built around how conditions present in white males. Autism research, until recently, used a 4:1 male-to-female ratio, assuming autism was primarily a "male" condition. ADHD research focused on hyperactive boys disrupting classrooms, missing the inattentive girls staring out windows, lost in their own worlds.

This bias creates a cascade of problems. Girls and women learn early to camouflage their differences. They watch other girls, copy their behaviors, and force themselves into neurotypical molds. By the time they seek help – usually after years of anxiety, depression, or burnout – their coping mechanisms are so refined that professionals see the mask, not the person beneath.

Research now shows that autistic girls and women present differently. They're more likely to have "social" special interests (like psychology or animals rather than trains). They mask their social difficulties through mimicry and scripting. They internalize their struggles, leading to anxiety and eating disorders rather than external behavioral problems.

The "female autism phenotype" overlaps significantly with BPD criteria. Both involve difficulty with identity (is it masking or identity disturbance?), emotional dysregulation (is it autistic meltdowns or BPD emotional instability?), and relationship struggles (is it social communication differences or fear of abandonment?). When you add ADHD to the mix – with its emotional dysregulation and executive dysfunction – the picture becomes even more complex.

Cultural Factors: The Missing Piece

Diagnostic disparities don't stop at gender. Research shows significant racial and ethnic disparities in diagnosis rates. Black and Latino children are diagnosed with autism an average of 2-3 years later than white children. Asian individuals often face the "model minority" stereotype, where their struggles are minimized or attributed to cultural differences rather than neurodevelopmental conditions.

Cultural factors affect how conditions manifest and how they're interpreted. In cultures that value social harmony, autistic traits might be seen as shyness or respect for authority. In cultures with different emotional expression norms, BPD might be misread as dramatic personality or attention-seeking. ADHD might be dismissed as laziness or lack of discipline in cultures that emphasize academic achievement.

These cultural blind spots mean that if you're not a white, middle-class male, your path to accurate diagnosis is likely longer and more complicated. You might have been told your struggles are personality flaws, cultural differences, or moral failings rather than neurological differences.

Language barriers add another layer of complexity. How do you describe executive dysfunction in a language that doesn't have words for it? How do you explain sensory overwhelm to a clinician who doesn't share your cultural understanding of sensory experiences?

These translation gaps – literal and cultural – contribute to misdiagnosis and delayed diagnosis.

The Trauma Tangle: When Everything Looks Like PTSD

Here's where things get really complicated: trauma changes the brain. And neurodivergent individuals are more likely to experience trauma. Studies show autistic individuals are 2-3 times more likely to experience PTSD. People with ADHD have higher rates of childhood trauma. And BPD is strongly associated with early relational trauma.

But trauma doesn't just co-occur with these conditions – it interweaves with them, creating presentations that can look entirely like PTSD or complex PTSD. Your sensory sensitivities might be attributed to hypervigilance. Your executive dysfunction might be seen as dissociation. Your emotional dysregulation might be viewed purely as trauma response.

The relationship between trauma and neurodevelopment is bidirectional. Being neurodivergent in a neurotypical world is inherently traumatic. You experience daily microaggressions, sensory assaults, and social rejections. This chronic stress shapes your nervous system, creating trauma responses layered on top of your innate neurological differences.

Many clinicians, seeing trauma in your history, stop there. They don't look underneath to see if there might be neurodevelopmental differences that both contributed to and were shaped by traumatic experiences. This is especially true for women and marginalized individuals, who are more likely to have their struggles attributed solely to trauma rather than considering neurological factors.

The Overlap Zone: Where Distinctions Blur

Let's examine specific areas where these conditions overlap so significantly that even experienced clinicians struggle to differentiate them:

Executive Function: All three conditions affect executive function, but differently. ADHD involves primary executive dysfunction – your brain's CEO is consistently unreliable. Autism involves executive dysfunction related to flexibility and transition difficulties. BPD involves executive function problems when emotionally dysregulated. When you have traits of all three, your executive function might vary wildly depending on emotional state, sensory environment, and routine disruption.

Emotional Regulation: ADHD includes rejection sensitive dysphoria – intense emotional pain from perceived rejection. Autism involves meltdowns and shutdowns from overwhelm. BPD involves intense, rapidly shifting emotions. But in real life, can you tell whether your emotional storm is RSD, autistic overwhelm, or BPD dysregulation? Often, it's all three, each triggering and amplifying the others.

Social Relationships: ADHD affects relationships through inattention, interrupting, and inconsistency. Autism affects relationships through communication differences and social confusion. BPD affects relationships through fear of abandonment and identity confusion. But when you experience all three, your relationships become a complex dance of missing cues, fearing rejection, and not knowing who you are with others.

Identity and Self: Perhaps the most confusing overlap is in identity. Autistic masking creates identity confusion – who are you beneath all the masks? ADHD's inconsistency makes it hard to maintain a stable sense of self. BPD involves core identity disturbance. When all three are present, the question "who am I?" becomes almost impossible to answer.

Diagnostic Tools: Why They Miss the Mark

Current diagnostic tools weren't designed for overlapping conditions. The Autism Diagnostic Observation Schedule (ADOS) might miss masked autism. ADHD rating scales might not capture internal hyperactivity. BPD assessments might pathologize autistic traits as personality problems.

Even worse, many tools have cut-off scores that exclude people who are "subclinical" in multiple areas but significantly impaired by the combination. You might score just below the autism threshold, just below the ADHD threshold, and just below the BPD threshold – but the cumulative effect of all three creates substantial disability.

Research shows that nearly 50% of women diagnosed with BPD score above the cut-off on autism screening tools. This isn't coincidence – it's evidence that our diagnostic categories might be artificial divisions in what's actually a spectrum of neurodevelopmental differences.

The solution isn't better tools – it's a better understanding of how these conditions interact. We need diagnostic processes that look at patterns across domains rather than checking boxes in isolated categories.

The Professional Perspective: Why Clinicians Struggle Too

Put yourself in a clinician's shoes for a moment. They have perhaps 45 minutes to assess you. They're using diagnostic criteria that don't fully capture masked presentations. They're working within a system that often requires a single primary diagnosis for insurance purposes. They might have limited training in neurodevelopmental conditions in adults, especially in their overlapping presentations.

Many clinicians default to what they know best. A psychiatrist might see everything through a mood disorder lens. A therapist trained in trauma might attribute everything to PTSD. A specialist in autism might miss the BPD traits. This isn't malicious – it's human nature to see what we're trained to see.

The pressure to diagnose quickly and treat efficiently means subtle presentations get missed. The quiet ADHD that looks like anxiety. The masked autism that looks like social anxiety. The internal BPD that looks like depression. These misdiagnoses aren't just incorrect labels – they lead to treatments that don't work and might even cause harm.

Building a Better Map: Integrated Understanding

What would diagnosis look like if we acknowledged the reality of overlapping conditions? First, it would involve longer assessments that examine patterns across the lifespan. It would include information from multiple sources – not just clinical observation but also self-report, family history, and real-world functioning.

An integrated diagnostic approach would look for patterns rather than isolated symptoms. Instead of asking "is this autism or BPD?" it would ask "how do autistic traits and BPD traits interact in this person?" Instead of forcing a primary diagnosis, it would acknowledge the reality of complex, overlapping presentations.

This approach would also consider cultural factors, gender presentation, and masking as central to diagnosis rather than complications to be ignored. It would recognize that someone can be "subclinical" in multiple areas but significantly impaired by the combination.

Your Personal Diagnostic Journey

Understanding why these conditions get confused empowers you to advocate for yourself. When you know that diagnostic criteria are imperfect, that bias exists, and that overlap is common, you can approach diagnosis differently.

You can prepare for assessments by documenting patterns across your lifetime, not just current symptoms. You can seek professionals who understand neurodevelopmental conditions in adults. You can ask specifically about their experience with overlapping conditions and masked presentations.

Most importantly, you can trust your own experience. If a diagnosis doesn't feel right, if treatments aren't working, if you relate more to lived experience accounts than clinical descriptions – trust that instinct. You know your inner world better than any professional who meets you for an hour.

Creating Your Own Understanding

While professional diagnosis can be validating and necessary for accessing support, your own understanding of your neurological differences is equally important. You can start building this understanding by examining patterns in your life:

Look at your childhood through a neurodevelopmental lens. Were there signs that got missed or misinterpreted? Did you develop coping mechanisms early that masked your differences? Were your struggles attributed to personality, laziness, or defiance rather than neurological differences?

Examine your current struggles without judgment. Where do you consistently struggle despite trying hard? What environments or situations consistently overwhelm you? What strategies have you developed that work, even if they seem unusual to others?

Consider your strengths alongside your challenges. Many neurodivergent individuals develop exceptional abilities in response to their differences. Your pattern recognition, creativity, intensity, or unique perspective might be the flip side of traits that get pathologized.

These ideas naturally lead us to explore the neuroscience behind these overlapping conditions. Understanding what's happening in your brain – the actual neurological differences underlying your experiences – can transform self-blame into self-compassion and confusion into clarity.

Chapter 3: Three Brains, Many Overlaps

The Neuroscience Made Simple

Your brain is having a conversation you can't hear. Right now, as you read this, billions of neurons are firing in patterns that shape how you experience the world. When you have ADHD, autism, and BPD traits, it's like your brain is speaking three different dialects of the same language – sometimes they harmonize, sometimes they clash, and sometimes they create entirely new meanings that nobody else seems to understand.

Understanding what's happening in your brain isn't about becoming a neuroscientist. It's about finally having an explanation for why certain things are so hard for you when they seem effortless for others. It's about replacing "what's wrong with me?" with "oh, that's why my brain does that."

Your Brain's Command Centers: A Guided Tour

Let's start with the basics – the key brain regions involved in ADHD, autism, and BPD. Think of your brain like a busy office building. The **prefrontal cortex** is the CEO's office, making executive decisions and planning ahead. The **amygdala** is the security system, always scanning for threats. The **hippocampus** is the filing system, storing and retrieving memories. And the **default mode network** is what happens during the lunch break – the background processing when you're not focused on specific tasks.

In ADHD, the CEO's office (prefrontal cortex) has an unreliable intercom system. Messages about what to prioritize get lost, delayed, or scrambled. The frontal-subcortical networks – the highways connecting the CEO to other departments – have inconsistent traffic flow. Sometimes information races through; sometimes it's gridlocked.

In autism, the whole building has different wiring. The sensory processing areas are either turned up to eleven or barely registering input. The social communication networks operate on different frequencies than the neurotypical standard. It's not broken – it's just built to different specifications.

In BPD, the security system (amygdala) is hypervigilant, and the emotion regulation circuits between the CEO's office and security are prone to short-circuiting. The hippocampus might be smaller – research shows 15-16% volume reduction in people with BPD, often linked to early trauma. When emotions flood the building, the CEO temporarily goes offline.

The ADHD Brain: Running on a Different Operating System

If neurotypical brains run on Windows, ADHD brains run on Linux – powerful, capable, but requiring different commands and producing unexpected results when you try to run standard programs. The key difference? Dopamine, your brain's motivation and reward chemical.

ADHD brains have differences in how they produce, release, and recycle dopamine. It's like having a smartphone with a battery that drains unpredictably and charges only with specific cables. This affects the frontal-subcortical networks – the pathways connecting your thinking brain to your doing brain.

Research has found reduced GABA in ADHD brains. GABA is your brain's brake pedal, the chemical that says "slow down, stop, think first." With less GABA, your brain struggles with inhibitory control. It's not that you don't want to stop interrupting or stay focused – your brain literally has worn brake pads.

These differences create a cascade of effects:

- Working memory becomes unreliable (where did I put my keys... while holding my keys)

- Time perception warps (5 minutes feels like an hour, an hour disappears in what feels like 5 minutes)

- Motivation requires higher stakes (regular rewards don't register; you need novelty or urgency)

- Emotional regulation becomes harder (feelings hit faster and stronger than your brain can process)

The Autistic Brain: Wired for Different Connections

Autism involves what researchers call "altered connectivity patterns" – some areas are hyper-connected while others are hypo-connected. Imagine a city where some neighborhoods have superhighways between them while others are connected only by winding country roads.

The sensory processing networks in autistic brains often have the volume turned up or down in unpredictable ways. A whisper might feel like shouting; a gentle touch might feel like sandpaper; or conversely, you might not notice you're hungry until you're about to faint. This isn't being "oversensitive" – your brain is literally processing sensory input differently.

Mirror neuron findings in autism are complex and often misunderstood. Mirror neurons help us automatically mimic and understand others' actions and emotions. In autism, these systems work differently – not broken, just different. You might need to consciously process what others do automatically, like manually operating a car that others drive automatically.

The autistic brain also shows differences in:

- Local vs. global processing (seeing details vs. big picture)

- Predictive processing (how your brain anticipates what comes next)

- Synaptic pruning (the process of refining neural connections)

- White matter organization (the brain's information highways)

These differences explain why you might notice patterns others miss, why unexpected changes feel catastrophic, and why social situations exhaust you – your brain is manually processing what others handle automatically.

The BPD Brain: When Emotions Override Everything

BPD involves what neuroscientists call fronto-limbic dysfunction. The frontal lobe (your rational, planning brain) and the limbic system (your emotional, survival brain) have a disrupted relationship. It's like having a smoke detector that goes off when you make toast – the alarm system works, but the calibration is off.

The amygdala in BPD tends to be hyperreactive. It sees danger everywhere, especially in relationships. A delayed text message registers as abandonment. A neutral facial expression reads as rejection. This isn't being "dramatic" – your brain is literally perceiving threat where others don't.

The HPA axis (hypothalamic-pituitary-adrenal axis) – your stress response system – is dysregulated in BPD. It's like being stuck in fight-or-flight mode, with cortisol flooding your system at the slightest trigger. This chronic stress actually changes brain structure, contributing to that hippocampal shrinkage mentioned earlier.

Key BPD brain differences include:

- Reduced prefrontal cortex activity during emotional tasks
- Increased amygdala reactivity to emotional stimuli
- Altered connectivity between emotion and control regions
- Differences in neurotransmitter systems (serotonin, dopamine, GABA)

When Three Conditions Collide: The Neurological Storm

Now here's where it gets really interesting – and complicated. When you have features of all three conditions, these brain differences don't just add up; they interact in complex ways.

Your ADHD dopamine dysregulation affects your autistic need for predictability – without enough dopamine, maintaining routines becomes even harder. Your autistic sensory sensitivities trigger your BPD emotional dysregulation. Your BPD fear of abandonment intensifies your ADHD rejection sensitivity. It's not three separate conditions; it's one complex neurological profile.

The overlapping neurotransmitter involvement creates compound effects:

- Dopamine (affected in ADHD and autism) influences emotional regulation

- Serotonin (affected in all three) impacts mood, sleep, and sensory processing

- GABA (reduced in ADHD and altered in autism) affects anxiety and inhibition

- Norepinephrine (dysregulated in ADHD and BPD) influences attention and stress response

These interactions explain why medication can be so tricky. Stimulants for ADHD might worsen anxiety. SSRIs for mood might worsen ADHD symptoms. What helps one aspect might aggravate another. Your brain isn't just running three programs – it's running three programs that constantly interact and modify each other.

The Plasticity Principle: Your Brain Can Change

Here's the hopeful part: neuroplasticity. Your brain can form new connections, strengthen different pathways, and even grow new neurons throughout your life. The differences in your brain aren't fixed destiny – they're your starting point.

Understanding your neurology isn't about accepting limitations; it's about working with your brain instead of against it. When you know your prefrontal cortex goes offline during emotional flooding, you can plan strategies for when you're calm. When you understand your sensory processing differences, you can create environments that support rather than overwhelm you.

Research shows that targeted interventions can actually change brain structure and function:

- Mindfulness practice increases prefrontal cortex density

- Therapy can reduce amygdala reactivity

- Exercise increases BDNF (brain-derived neurotrophic factor), supporting neural growth

- Sensory integration work can help regulate processing differences

Making Sense of Your Unique Wiring

Your brain might process information differently, but different doesn't mean defective. That hyperfocus that makes you lose track of time? That's your brain's ability to achieve flow states others only dream of. That emotional intensity that feels overwhelming? It's also what allows you to experience joy, creativity, and connection deeply.

The sensory sensitivity that makes clothes shopping torture also lets you notice subtle beauty others miss. The hypervigilance that exhausts you also makes you incredibly perceptive about others' emotions. The executive dysfunction that makes daily tasks difficult is often paired with innovative thinking and creative problem-solving.

Understanding your neurology helps you:

- Stop blaming yourself for brain-based differences

- Identify strategies that work with your wiring

- Explain your needs to others with scientific backing

- Recognize when you need support versus when you need different strategies

Brain Difference Doesn't Mean Brain Deficit: Reframing Exercise

Take a moment to reframe your brain differences:

1. List three things your brain struggles with

2. For each struggle, identify a potential strength or advantage it might create

3. Consider: How might this difference be adaptive in certain contexts?

For example:

- Struggle: Emotional intensity

- Potential strength: Deep empathy and connection capacity

- Adaptive context: Crisis support, creative fields, advocacy work

Understanding My Sensory-Emotional-Executive Profile: Assessment

Rate each area from 1 (significant challenges) to 5 (area of strength):

Sensory Processing:

- Visual sensitivity (lights, patterns, movement)

- Auditory processing (noises, conversations, background sounds)

- Tactile sensitivity (textures, temperatures, touch)

- Interoception (hunger, thirst, bathroom needs, internal sensations)

Emotional Regulation:

- Identifying emotions as they arise
- Tolerating emotional discomfort
- Recovering from emotional overwhelm
- Expressing emotions appropriately

Executive Function:

- Starting tasks (initiation)
- Switching between tasks (flexibility)
- Organizing and planning
- Working memory
- Impulse control

Look at your pattern. Where do you see overlaps between sensory, emotional, and executive challenges? These intersection points are where the three conditions might be interacting in your brain.

Having mapped this terrain of your neurological landscape, you're ready to explore how these brain differences play out in daily life through executive function, emotional regulation, and sensory processing.

Chapter 4: Executive Function, Emotional Regulation, and Sensory Processing

You wake up with the best intentions. Today will be different. You'll follow your schedule, stay calm during that meeting, and finally tackle that project. Three hours later, you're somehow reorganizing your entire closet while the project remains untouched, you're overwhelmed by your coworker's perfume, and you're fighting back tears over a comment that "shouldn't" bother you.

This isn't failure. This is what happens when executive dysfunction, emotional dysregulation, and sensory processing differences team up to hijack your day. When you understand how these three systems interact – especially when ADHD, autism, and BPD overlap – you can stop fighting yourself and start working with your brain's unique operating system.

Executive Function: Your Brain's Air Traffic Controller

Executive function is like air traffic control for your brain – coordinating multiple flights (thoughts, actions, emotions) to land safely without crashing into each other. When it works well, you can plan your day, switch between tasks, remember what you're doing, and stop yourself from doing things you'll regret.

But here's the thing: ADHD, autism, and BPD each affect executive function differently, and when you have traits of all three, your air traffic control tower is dealing with three different weather systems simultaneously.

ADHD Executive Dysfunction is like having an air traffic controller who randomly goes on coffee breaks. Sometimes they're hyper-focused on one plane while ignoring others. Sometimes they're trying to land fifty planes at once. The core issues include:

- Task initiation paralysis (staring at the task but unable to start)

- Time blindness (losing three hours to something that should take twenty minutes)

- Working memory gaps (walking into a room and forgetting why)

- Priority confusion (organizing paperclips while the house burns down)

Autistic Executive Dysfunction involves rigidity and transition difficulties. Your air traffic controller has very specific protocols and panics when planes need to change course. This shows up as:

- Difficulty with unexpected changes

- Struggling to switch between activities

- Getting stuck on specific ways of doing things

- Needing extra processing time for new instructions

BPD-Related Executive Dysfunction happens when emotions flood the control tower. When you're emotionally dysregulated, your executive function temporarily goes offline. You might:

- Make impulsive decisions during emotional storms

- Struggle to access coping strategies when triggered

- Find planning impossible when fearing abandonment

- Experience cognitive fog during identity confusion

When all three overlap, you get compound executive dysfunction that varies based on emotional state, sensory environment, and routine disruption. Monday's strategy might not work on Tuesday. What helps in the morning might fail by afternoon.

The Reality of Living with Triple Executive Dysfunction

Let's look at how this plays out in real life. A college student with overlapping traits sits down to study. Their ADHD brain struggles to start. Their autistic brain needs the perfect setup – right lighting, right temperature, right background noise. Their BPD brain interprets their struggle as proof they're worthless, triggering emotional dysregulation that shuts down executive function entirely.

Or consider a parent trying to manage household tasks. The ADHD makes them forget what they're doing mid-task. The autism makes transitioning between tasks feel impossible. The BPD emotional sensitivity means a partner's innocent comment derails their entire system. They end up exhausted, having started twenty things and finished nothing.

This isn't laziness or lack of trying. Your brain is literally working with different wiring, and expecting it to function like a neurotypical brain is like expecting a Mac to run Windows software without an emulator.

Emotional Regulation: When Three Alarm Systems Overlap

Emotional regulation is your ability to recognize, understand, and manage your emotional responses. Think of it like a thermostat – sensing the temperature and adjusting accordingly. But what happens when you have three different thermostats all trying to control the same system?

ADHD Emotional Dysregulation includes rejection sensitive dysphoria (RSD) – intense physical and emotional pain from perceived rejection or criticism. It's not just feeling sad when someone criticizes you; it's feeling like you've been physically punched. ADHD emotions also tend to be:

- Quickly triggered

- Intensely felt

- Short-lived (when not complicated by rumination)

- Hard to hide or control

Autistic Emotional Dysregulation often stems from:

- Sensory overload triggering meltdowns

- Communication frustrations building to explosion

- Change or uncertainty causing overwhelming anxiety

- Alexithymia (difficulty identifying and describing emotions)

- Delayed emotional processing (realizing you're upset hours later)

BPD Emotional Dysregulation is characterized by:

- Emotions shifting rapidly and unpredictably

- Emotional responses disproportionate to triggers

- Difficulty self-soothing once activated

- Emotions feeling like facts rather than temporary states

- Chronic emptiness punctuated by emotional storms

When these three systems overlap, you might experience emotional cascades. A sensory trigger (autism) leads to frustration, which triggers rejection sensitivity (ADHD), which activates abandonment fears (BPD), creating an emotional avalanche that takes hours or days to recover from.

The Emotional Weather Pattern of Your Day

Imagine tracking your emotional weather throughout a typical day. Morning starts with sensory overwhelm from getting ready (autism), creating baseline irritability. A work email triggers RSD (ADHD), sending you into an emotional spiral. This emotional dysregulation makes you snap at a friend, triggering abandonment fears (BPD) and shame that perpetuates the cycle.

You're not "too emotional" or "overreacting." You're managing three different emotional regulation systems that sometimes work against each other. It's like trying to drive a car where the gas pedal, brake, and steering wheel each have their own agenda.

Sensory Processing: Your Neural Filter System

Sensory processing is how your nervous system receives and responds to sensory information. Most people have automatic filters that screen out irrelevant sensory input. But when you have ADHD, autism, and BPD traits, your filters work differently.

ADHD Sensory Processing involves:

- Sensory seeking behaviors (needing intense input to feel regulated)

- Hyposensitivity requiring stronger stimuli to register

- Attention-related filtering problems (can't tune out background noise)

- Fluctuating sensory needs based on dopamine levels

Autistic Sensory Processing includes:

- Hypersensitivity to specific stimuli (textures, sounds, lights)

- Hyposensitivity in some areas requiring more input

- Sensory overload leading to shutdown or meltdown

- Difficulty with interoception (internal body signals)

- Synesthesia or unusual sensory experiences

BPD Sensory Processing is less discussed but includes:

- Emotional states affecting sensory tolerance

- Dissociation altering sensory perception

- Using sensory input for emotional regulation (or dysregulation)

- Hypersensitivity to emotional atmospheres and others' moods

The overlap creates a sensory experience that's constantly shifting. Your tolerance for sensory input might change based on:

- Emotional state (BPD)
- Attention and energy levels (ADHD)
- Accumulated sensory load (autism)
- Time of day and routine disruption (all three)

Interoception: The Hidden Eighth Sense

Interoception – awareness of internal body signals – deserves special attention because it's affected by all three conditions and rarely discussed. It's your ability to notice hunger, thirst, need for the bathroom, temperature, pain, and emotional sensations in your body.

Poor interoception means you might:

- Not notice hunger until you're shaking
- Forget to use the bathroom for hours
- Not recognize emotional buildup until explosion
- Struggle to identify what you're feeling
- Miss early warning signs of overload

This isn't absent-mindedness – your brain literally processes internal signals differently. When you add alexithymia (common in autism), emotional dysregulation (all three conditions), and attention difficulties (ADHD), you get a perfect storm of interoceptive confusion.

The Compound Effect: When Systems Interact

Here's where understanding gets crucial: these systems don't operate independently. They're constantly influencing each other in feedback loops that can either stabilize or destabilize your entire system.

Consider this cascade:

1. Poor interoception means you don't notice you're hungry
2. Low blood sugar affects executive function
3. Executive dysfunction prevents task completion
4. Task failure triggers emotional dysregulation
5. Emotional flooding increases sensory sensitivity
6. Sensory overload further impairs executive function
7. The cycle continues and amplifies

Or this one:

1. Sensory overload from a busy environment
2. Depletes executive function resources trying to filter
3. Can't access emotional regulation strategies
4. Emotional dysregulation makes sensory input worse
5. Complete system overwhelm and shutdown

Understanding these cascades helps you identify intervention points. Maybe you can't prevent sensory overload, but you can notice early signs and reduce demands on executive function. Maybe you can't stop emotional dysregulation, but you can create sensory comfort to prevent additional overwhelm.

Building Your Personal Operating Manual

Every brain is different, and your combination of traits creates a unique profile. Building your personal operating manual means mapping:

Your Executive Function Pattern:

- When is it strongest? (time of day, environment, emotional state)

- What depletes it fastest? (transitions, decisions, sensory input)

- What restores it? (movement, quiet, stimulation, rest)

Your Emotional Regulation Map:

- What are your triggers? (rejection, change, sensory, social)

- What are your early warning signs? (body sensations, thoughts, behaviors)

- What helps you regulate? (movement, pressure, temperature, connection)

Your Sensory Profile:

- What sensory input calms you? (weight, movement, sound, texture)

- What overwhelms you? (lights, sounds, textures, crowds)

- How does this change based on other factors?

Executive Function Assessment Tool

Rate your executive function in different contexts (1 = severe difficulty, 5 = works well):

Morning vs. Evening:

- Task initiation

- Planning and organization

- Working memory

- Cognitive flexibility

- Impulse control

Calm vs. Stressed:

- Task initiation
- Planning and organization
- Working memory
- Cognitive flexibility
- Impulse control

Alone vs. With Others:

- Task initiation
- Planning and organization
- Working memory
- Cognitive flexibility
- Impulse control

Notice patterns. When does your executive function work best? What conditions support it?

Emotional Regulation Strategies Chart

Create your personalized chart:

Preventive Strategies (use when calm):

- ADHD: Regular movement, stimulation breaks, RSD preparation
- Autism: Routine maintenance, sensory regulation, transition planning
- BPD: Attachment security building, identity affirmation, distress tolerance practice

In-the-Moment Strategies (use during dysregulation):

- ADHD: Physical movement, intense sensory input, external validation

- Autism: Reduction of demands, sensory comfort, routine restoration

- BPD: Self-soothing, connection with safe person, grounding exercises

Recovery Strategies (use after dysregulation):

- ADHD: Self-compassion, perspective-taking, energy restoration

- Autism: Sensory recovery, routine re-establishment, processing time

- BPD: Identity restoration, relationship repair, emotional validation

Practical Integration: Making It All Work

Understanding these three systems and their interactions isn't just academic – it's the key to creating a life that works with your brain rather than against it. This might mean:

- Scheduling high executive function tasks for your best times

- Building sensory regulation into your daily routine

- Creating emotional regulation plans while calm

- Recognizing cascade patterns early

- Having different strategies for different states

- Accepting that your needs vary day to day

With these pieces in place, you're ready to explore how these neurological differences manifest in specific diagnostic presentations. Understanding your brain's infrastructure helps make sense of the symptoms that might have confused you and professionals alike.

Chapter 5: Is It ADHD?

Understanding Attention, Impulsivity, and Hyperactivity

You know that feeling when someone asks if you have ADHD and you start explaining, but halfway through you forget what you were saying, interrupt yourself with three different thoughts, and then realize you've been clicking your pen for the past five minutes? Yeah, that might be worth exploring.

ADHD isn't just about being hyper or distracted. It's a fundamental difference in how your brain processes information, manages time, and regulates everything from emotions to energy. And here's what makes it even more complex – ADHD looks radically different depending on your age, gender, and what other conditions might be dancing alongside it.

The Three Faces of ADHD That Nobody Talks About

Most people think ADHD comes in two flavors: hyperactive or inattentive. But reality is messier. There are actually three presentations, and they can shift throughout your life like a shape-changing puzzle that refuses to stay still.

Inattentive presentation is the daydreamer, the one staring out the window while life happens around them. But calling it "inattentive" is misleading – you're not lacking attention, you're drowning in it. Every thought, sound, and sensation gets equal billing in your brain. You might hyperfocus on reorganizing your bookshelf for six hours while your work deadline whooshes by. Your attention isn't deficit; it's just playing by different rules.

Hyperactive-impulsive presentation isn't always the stereotypical bouncing-off-walls kid. In adults, especially women, it often shows up as internal restlessness. Your mind races while your body stays still. You interrupt people not because you're rude but because if you don't say the thought right now, it'll disappear forever. You make impulsive decisions – quit jobs, start relationships, buy things you don't need – because in that moment, the impulse feels like the only truth that exists.

Combined presentation is where most adults with ADHD eventually land. You get the complete package – the mental fog and the mental NASCAR race, the paralysis and the impulsivity, the hyperfocus and the inability to focus on anything that matters. It's exhausting, contradictory, and probably why people keep telling you you're "too much" and "not enough" at the same time.

Rejection Sensitive Dysphoria: The ADHD Secret Nobody Mentions

Here's something that affects 99% of people with ADHD but rarely makes it into diagnostic conversations: Rejection Sensitive Dysphoria (RSD). It's not just being sensitive to criticism – it's experiencing perceived rejection as physical pain. Your nervous system responds to a critical email the same way it would to being punched.

RSD means you might:

- Replay conversations for hours, analyzing every word for signs of rejection

- Avoid trying new things because the possibility of failure feels unbearable

- People-please to the point of exhaustion

- Have emotional reactions that seem "over the top" to others

- Create elaborate mental scenarios of how people probably hate you

This isn't weakness or drama. Your ADHD brain literally processes emotional pain differently. The same neurological differences that affect your attention also affect how you experience social and emotional feedback. When someone says "we need to talk," your brain might interpret it as "you're about to be abandoned forever."

Executive Dysfunction: When Your Brain's CEO Goes AWOL

Executive function is your brain's management system. With ADHD, it's like having a CEO who's brilliant but completely unreliable. Sometimes they show up and everything runs smoothly. Sometimes they disappear for three days without warning.

Executive dysfunction in ADHD affects:

- **Working memory** – Information falls out of your brain like water through a sieve

- **Task initiation** – You know what needs doing but can't make yourself start

- **Time awareness** – Five minutes and five hours feel identical until suddenly they don't

- **Emotional regulation** – Feelings hit like tsunamis before you can process them

- **Cognitive flexibility** – Switching between tasks feels like changing dimensions

- **Planning and prioritization** – Everything feels equally urgent and equally impossible

The frustrating part? Your executive function can work perfectly when conditions are right – novel, interesting, urgent, or challenging tasks might activate hyperfocus. But ask you to do something boring but important? Your brain's CEO has left the building.

The Gender Gap Nobody Wants to Admit

Women with ADHD are diagnosed on average 3.9 years later than men. Why? Because ADHD research, diagnostic criteria, and cultural expectations were built around how it presents in boys. Girls learn early to mask their symptoms, internalize their hyperactivity, and compensate until they can't anymore.

In women and girls, ADHD often looks like:

- Anxiety and depression (which get treated while ADHD gets missed)

- Eating disorders (dopamine seeking through food or control)

- Perfectionism covering up executive dysfunction

- Chronic overwhelm dismissed as "just stress"

- Relationship chaos attributed to personality rather than neurology

- Physical hyperactivity channeled into socially acceptable fidgeting

The internal hyperactivity is real but invisible. Your thoughts race, your emotions spiral, your mental energy burns like a wildfire, but outside you look calm. You've learned to sit still while your insides vibrate at frequencies that could shatter glass. This isn't "mild" ADHD – it's ADHD with a degree in masking.

ADHD Across Your Lifetime: It Doesn't Go Away, It Shape-Shifts

Childhood ADHD might mean trouble in school, but adult ADHD means trouble with... everything. Work, relationships, self-care, finances, health – ADHD touches every aspect of adult life in ways nobody prepared you for.

In your 20s, ADHD might look like:

- Starting college majors you never finish

- Intense but short-lived relationships

- Impulsive decisions that seem like adventures

- Time blindness that makes you chronically late
- Hyperfocus that helps you excel in areas of interest

In your 30s and 40s, it might shift to:

- Parenting challenges when you can barely parent yourself
- Career struggles despite obvious intelligence
- Relationship patterns you can see but can't seem to change
- Mounting shame about "still" struggling with "basic" things
- Health issues from years of stress and poor self-care

In your 50s and beyond, especially if undiagnosed:

- Decades of accumulated shame and self-blame
- Coping mechanisms that stopped working
- Grief over the life you might have had with earlier support
- But also: self-acceptance and wisdom about your brain
- Freedom to stop masking and start accommodating

ADHD doesn't disappear with age – it just changes costumes.

The Co-Occurring Conditions Club

ADHD rarely travels alone. It usually brings friends, and those friends complicate everything. Understanding these co-occurrences helps explain why your ADHD might look different from someone else's.

Common companions include:

- **Anxiety disorders** (50% of adults with ADHD)
- **Depression** (up to 30%)
- **Autism** (30-50% overlap)

- **Learning disabilities** (30-50%)

- **Substance use disorders** (self-medication is real)

- **Sleep disorders** (75% have sleep issues)

- **Bipolar disorder** (20% of people with bipolar have ADHD)

- **Borderline Personality Disorder** (30% of people with ADHD)

These aren't just complications – they're clues. If you have ADHD plus anxiety, your treatment needs to address both. If you have ADHD plus autism, strategies that work for pure ADHD might backfire spectacularly.

The Reality Check: What Living with ADHD Actually Means

Let's get specific about daily life with ADHD. You wake up with seventeen thoughts already racing. You had plans for today, but your brain has other ideas. You sit down to work and suddenly it's three hours later and you've researched the entire history of medieval farming techniques instead of answering emails.

You lose things that are literally in your hand. You forget appointments while looking at your calendar. You buy the same thing twice because you forgot you bought it, then forget to return the extra. You have fourteen half-finished projects and starting a new one feels easier than finishing an old one.

Relationships are complicated because you interrupt, forget important dates, and zone out during conversations, but you also love intensely, think creatively, and bring energy that lights up rooms. You're reliable in crisis but struggle with routine maintenance. You give amazing advice you can't follow yourself.

The medication question looms large. Stimulants might help but come with side effects and stigma. Non-stimulant options exist but work differently. Some people thrive on medication; others find non-medication strategies more sustainable. There's no universal answer, only what works for your brain in your life.

Building Your ADHD Understanding Toolkit

Living with ADHD means becoming an expert on your own brain. This means tracking patterns:

When does your attention work best? Morning, evening, after exercise, with background noise, in silence? What depletes it fastest? What restores it?

What triggers your RSD? Certain people, situations, times of day? What helps you recover? Movement, music, talking it out, time alone?

Which executive functions fail first when you're stressed? Which ones are most reliable? What scaffolding helps? Apps, alarms, accountability partners, visual cues?

ADHD Symptom Tracker: A Week in Your Brain

For one week, track:

Morning:

- Energy level (1-10)
- Focus capacity (1-10)
- Emotional regulation (1-10)
- What helped or hurt?

Afternoon:

- Energy level (1-10)
- Focus capacity (1-10)
- Emotional regulation (1-10)
- What helped or hurt?

Evening:

- Energy level (1-10)

- Focus capacity (1-10)

- Emotional regulation (1-10)

- What helped or hurt?

Look for patterns. When do you function best? What consistently helps or hinders?

The Unspoken Truth About ADHD

Here's what professionals might not tell you: ADHD involves real suffering. The suicide risk is 30% higher than the general population. Not because ADHD makes you suicidal, but because living in a world not built for your brain takes a toll. The constant criticism, the shame, the exhaustion of trying to function in systems that don't accommodate you – it adds up.

But here's the other truth: ADHD also involves real gifts. Creativity, intuition, the ability to see connections others miss, energy that can move mountains when directed, hyperfocus that produces brilliance, and a different perspective that the world desperately needs.

Understanding ADHD isn't about fixing yourself. It's about recognizing that your brain has a different operating system – not better or worse, just different. With that understanding comes the power to stop fighting your nature and start working with it.

With this foundation laid within you about ADHD's complex presentation, let's explore another piece of the puzzle – autism and its hidden manifestations.

Chapter 6: Is It Autism?

Unmasking the Hidden Spectrum

So you've made it to adulthood thinking you're just quirky, sensitive, or maybe a bit intense, and then someone mentions autism. Your first thought might be "but I make eye contact" or "I have friends" or "I'm not like Rain Man." Here's the thing – autism in adults, especially those who've learned to mask, looks nothing like the stereotypes.

The autism spectrum isn't a line from "less autistic" to "more autistic." It's more like a color wheel where each person has their own unique mix of traits, intensities, and presentations. And if you've made it to adulthood undiagnosed, you've probably become an expert at hiding your autistic traits – even from yourself.

High-Masking Autism: The Performance That's Killing You

Masking is what happens when autistic people consciously or unconsciously hide their autistic traits to fit into neurotypical society. It's the script you run in social situations, the constant monitoring of your body language, the exhausting performance of "normal" that leaves you drained.

The Camouflaging Autistic Traits Questionnaire (CAT-Q) identifies three types of masking:

Compensation – You actively compensate for social difficulties. You might maintain eye contact even though it's painful, force yourself through small talk using scripts, or study social rules like an anthropologist studying a foreign culture.

Masking – You hide your autistic traits. You suppress stims, force yourself to tolerate sensory discomfort, hide your special interests, and present a "normal" facade that takes tremendous energy to maintain.

Assimilation – You try to fit in with neurotypical peers. You copy others' behaviors, interests, and communication styles. You might not even know who you really are anymore because you've been playing roles for so long.

Research shows that high-masking autistic adults, especially women and marginalized folks, often don't get diagnosed until their 30s, 40s, or later. By then, you've usually collected a handful of mental health diagnoses – anxiety, depression, borderline personality disorder – that treat the symptoms of living as an unidentified autistic person but miss the root cause.

Social Communication vs. Social Motivation: The Misunderstanding That Changes Everything

Here's a revolutionary thought: most autistic people want social connection. The stereotype of autistic people not caring about others? Complete nonsense. The difference isn't in motivation – it's in communication styles.

Neurotypical social communication relies heavily on:

- Nonverbal cues that might be invisible to you
- Implied meanings you're supposed to "just know"
- Social hierarchies that seem arbitrary
- Small talk that feels pointless and exhausting
- Flexible social rules that change without warning

Autistic social communication tends to involve:

- Direct, honest communication (which gets labeled as "rude")
- Information sharing as connection (infodumping about special interests)

- Parallel play and companionship without constant interaction

- Deep, meaningful conversations over surface-level chat

- Consistent social rules that make logical sense

You might deeply want connection but struggle with neurotypical social expectations. You might have learned to perform social interaction without understanding why you're doing what you're doing. It's like speaking a second language where you know the words but not the music.

Monotropic Attention and Special Interests: Your Brain's Superpower

Monotropism is an attention theory that explains a lot about autistic thinking. Instead of spreading attention across multiple channels (polytropic), autistic brains tend to focus intensely on fewer things at once (monotropic). It's not a deficit – it's a different attention strategy.

This explains:

- Why transitions are so hard (shifting that intense focus takes enormous energy)

- Why interruptions feel catastrophic (you lose the entire attention tunnel)

- Why you might not notice hunger, thirst, or bathroom needs when focused

- Why multitasking might be impossible or exhausting

- Why special interests feel so compelling and necessary

Special interests aren't just hobbies. They're where your monotropic attention finds its home. They might be traditionally "autistic" (trains, computers) or completely unexpected (fashion, reality TV, spreadsheets). The key is the intensity and the way engaging with them regulates your nervous system.

Special interests serve multiple functions:

- Emotional regulation when overwhelmed

- Predictable source of joy and competence

- Social connection point with others who share the interest

- Career paths when you're lucky enough to monetize them

- Identity anchors in a confusing world

Sensory Differences: Living in a Different Perceptual Universe

Sensory processing differences are now part of autism diagnostic criteria, finally acknowledging what autistic people have always known – we literally experience the world differently.

This might mean:

- **Hypersensitivity** – Lights too bright, sounds too loud, textures unbearable

- **Hyposensitivity** – Not noticing pain, temperature, or internal signals

- **Sensory seeking** – Craving intense input like pressure, movement, or specific textures

- **Sensory avoiding** – Organizing life around preventing sensory overwhelm

- **Fluctuating sensitivity** – What's tolerable changes based on stress, energy, time of day

You might have spent your life being called "too sensitive" or "difficult" when really your nervous system is processing sensory information differently. That tag in your shirt isn't just annoying – it might feel like torture. The fluorescent lights aren't just unpleasant – they might make thinking impossible.

The Female Autism Phenotype: Why Women Get Missed

The "female autism phenotype" describes how autism often presents differently in women and girls (though people of any gender can have this presentation). These differences explain why so many women don't get diagnosed until adulthood.

Common features include:

- Better superficial social mimicry

- Special interests in people, psychology, or animals rather than objects

- Internalizing difficulties rather than externalizing

- Using imagination and fantasy as coping mechanisms

- Higher rates of eating disorders and anxiety

- More sophisticated masking strategies

- Interests that appear more socially acceptable

This isn't "mild" autism – it's autism with advanced camouflaging. The cost of this masking is enormous. By adulthood, many women have developed anxiety disorders, eating disorders, depression, and chronic exhaustion from decades of performing neurotypicality.

Autistic Burnout: When the Mask Becomes Too Heavy

Autistic burnout happens when the cumulative effect of masking, sensory overload, and living in a neurotypical world becomes too much. It's not regular burnout – it's a neurological crisis that can last months or years.

Autistic burnout might include:

- Loss of skills you previously had (speech, executive function, self-care)

- Increased sensory sensitivity

- Inability to mask anymore

- Severe exhaustion that rest doesn't fix

- Increased meltdowns or shutdowns

- Loss of ability to tolerate things you previously managed

Many adults seek autism assessment during or after burnout. The mask finally cracks, and what's underneath can't be hidden anymore. This is often terrifying but also liberating – you finally have permission to stop pretending.

Recovery from autistic burnout requires:

- Reducing masking and social demands

- Sensory regulation and accommodation

- Accepting support and accommodations

- Reconnecting with authentic interests and needs

- Time – often much more than expected

The DSM-5-TR Finally Gets It (Sort Of)

The updated DSM-5-TR includes a crucial addition: symptoms "may be masked by learned strategies in later life." This single sentence validates what adult-diagnosed autistics have been saying forever – just because you've learned to compensate doesn't mean you're not autistic.

But diagnosis is still challenging because:

- Most tools were designed for children

- Masking isn't well understood by many professionals

- Childhood history might be hard to obtain

- Co-occurring conditions complicate the picture

- Cultural and gender biases persist

Getting an accurate autism diagnosis as an adult often requires:

48

- Finding a specialist in adult autism

- Preparing extensive documentation of traits

- Including childhood history when possible

- Being prepared to advocate for yourself

- Sometimes seeking multiple opinions

Living While Autistic: The Reality Beyond Diagnosis

Whether formally diagnosed or self-identified, understanding your autistic traits changes everything. Suddenly, your whole life makes sense. The sensory issues, the social confusion, the intense interests, the need for routine – it all fits together.

Daily life as an autistic adult might mean:

- Planning everything around sensory tolerance

- Needing recovery time after social interaction

- Having scripts for common conversations

- Struggling with things others find simple (phone calls, grocery stores)

- Excelling at things others find difficult (pattern recognition, deep focus)

- Feeling like an anthropologist studying human behavior

- Finding your people in autistic communities

Work can be particularly challenging. Open offices are sensory nightmares. Team meetings drain your social battery. Unwritten rules and office politics are inscrutable. But you might also bring unique strengths – attention to detail, innovative thinking, deep expertise, and reliability in routine tasks.

Building Your Autism Understanding

Understanding your autism isn't about limitations – it's about finally having the user manual for your brain. This means identifying:

Your sensory profile: What overwhelms you? What soothes you? What do you seek? What do you avoid? How does this change throughout the day?

Your social capacity: How much interaction can you handle? What types drain you least? How long does recovery take? What accommodations help?

Your communication style: Do you prefer written over verbal? Direct over indirect? Information sharing over emotion sharing? How can you get your needs met?

Your regulation needs: What routines keep you stable? What interests regulate you? What environments support you? What changes destabilize you?

Autism Traits Inventory: Mapping Your Neurodivergence

Consider these areas:

Sensory:

- Which senses are most sensitive?
- What are your seeking behaviors?
- What are your avoiding behaviors?
- How does stress affect sensitivity?

Social:

- What social situations are hardest?
- What masking strategies do you use?
- How much social interaction feels right?
- What types of connection work best?

Routine and Change:

- Which routines are essential?
- How do you handle unexpected changes?
- What transitions are hardest?
- What helps with flexibility?

Communication:

- Do you struggle with nonverbal cues?
- Is phone communication harder than text?
- Do you take language literally?
- How do you handle implied meanings?

The Hidden Gifts of Autism

While we talk about struggles, let's not forget – autism comes with genuine cognitive differences that can be advantages:

- **Pattern recognition** that borders on prescient
- **Attention to detail** others completely miss
- **Loyalty and honesty** that's refreshing in a world of social games
- **Deep knowledge** in areas of interest
- **Innovative thinking** from processing information differently
- **Sensory perception** that notices beauty others miss
- **Genuine connection** when you find your people

The world needs autistic minds. Your different perspective, your refusal to follow arbitrary social rules, your deep dives into specific topics, your sensory sensitivity – these aren't just quirks to be tolerated but valuable differences that contribute to human diversity.

As these patterns become visible and your understanding of autism deepens, you're ready to explore another piece of the diagnostic puzzle – the quiet, internal presentation of borderline personality disorder.

Chapter 7: Is It Quiet BPD?

When Emotions Turn Inward

Most people think borderline personality disorder means dramatic outbursts, suicide attempts, and hospital visits. But there's another presentation that flies completely under the radar – quiet BPD, where all that emotional intensity turns inward instead of outward. You're not throwing things or screaming. You're silently imploding while maintaining a perfectly normal facade. The storm rages, but only you can hear it.

If you've been told you have anxiety, depression, or even autism when something deeper feels wrong, quiet BPD might be the missing piece. It shares so many features with other conditions that even experienced clinicians miss it. But understanding quiet BPD – especially how it interacts with ADHD and autism – can finally explain why you feel like you're drowning in emotions nobody else can see.

Quiet BPD vs. Classic BPD: Same Storm, Different Expression

Quiet BPD involves the same core features as "classic" BPD – fear of abandonment, identity disturbance, emotional dysregulation, unstable relationships. But instead of externalizing these struggles, you internalize everything. Think of it like the difference between a volcano and a sinkhole. Both involve massive geological disruption, but one explodes outward while the other collapses inward.

In quiet BPD, the symptoms manifest as:

Self-directed anger instead of outward rage. When triggered, you don't lash out at others – you tear yourself apart internally. The fury you feel gets directed at yourself through vicious self-criticism, self-harm, or self-sabotage. Others might not even know you're angry.

People-pleasing instead of conflict. Rather than the push-pull dynamic of classic BPD relationships, you might become whoever others need you to be. You're so terrified of abandonment that you abandon yourself first, shapeshifting to avoid any possibility of rejection.

Dissociation instead of visible dysregulation. When emotions become overwhelming, you don't explode – you disappear. You might look calm on the outside while being completely disconnected from your body, floating somewhere above yourself watching life happen.

Silent suffering instead of help-seeking. While classic BPD might involve frequent crisis calls or emergency room visits, quiet BPD means suffering alone. You might be actively suicidal while telling everyone you're fine. The idea of burdening others with your pain is unbearable.

Emotional implosion instead of explosion. All that intensity doesn't go away – it just goes inward. You might spend hours in mental loops of self-hatred, replay every social interaction for signs of rejection, or punish yourself for emotions you "shouldn't" have.

The quiet presentation often develops in environments where emotional expression was dangerous or punished. Maybe you learned early that showing distress led to worse outcomes. Maybe you were the "good" child who had to hold everything together. Maybe your survival depended on being invisible.

Identity Disturbance vs. Masking Confusion: Who Are You Really?

One of the most confusing aspects of quiet BPD is the identity disturbance – not knowing who you really are. But wait, doesn't that sound exactly like autistic masking? Or ADHD inconsistency? How do you tell the difference?

BPD identity disturbance feels like you're empty at the core. You're not hiding a true self; you genuinely don't know if there IS a true self. You might:

- Feel like a different person with different people
- Adopt others' interests, values, even mannerisms completely
- Feel existentially empty when alone
- Change fundamental beliefs based on who you're with
- Feel like you're performing "human" rather than being human

Autistic masking involves hiding your authentic self to fit in. There IS a real you underneath – you just learned it wasn't acceptable. The difference:

- You know what you like when you're alone
- Your core values remain even if hidden
- Unmasking feels like relief, not emptiness
- You're translating yourself, not shape-shifting
- Special interests remain consistent even if hidden

ADHD inconsistency comes from executive dysfunction and dopamine-seeking. Your interests might change rapidly, but you're not empty:

- Interest changes follow dopamine, not people
- Core self remains even as expressions change
- Alone time might be scattered but not empty
- You forget things, not fundamental self

The reality? If you have all three conditions, these experiences layer and interact. You might have autistic masking that turned into BPD-like identity confusion after years of not knowing who you were allowed to be. Your ADHD might make it harder to maintain consistent sense of self. Untangling them might be less important than understanding how they work together in your specific experience.

Attachment Patterns and the Terror of Abandonment

The fear of abandonment in quiet BPD isn't just worry about being left – it's complete existential terror. But unlike classic BPD, where this might lead to frantic efforts to avoid abandonment, quiet BPD often involves preemptive self-abandonment. You leave first, emotionally if not physically, to avoid the pain of being left.

Your attachment pattern might look like:

Anxious-avoidant hybrid: You desperately want closeness but are terrified of it. You might get close to someone, then panic and withdraw. Unlike pure avoidant attachment, you're not indifferent – you're in agony, wanting connection but believing you'll destroy it.

Emotional fusion alternating with detachment: You might merge completely with someone, losing all boundaries, then suddenly feel suffocated and need complete distance. This isn't the same as autistic need for alone time – it's driven by terror of both abandonment and engulfment.

Preemptive rejection: You might end relationships that are going well because you "know" they'll eventually leave. Better to be the one who leaves than the one who's left. You might sabotage good things because happiness feels like a setup for devastating loss.

Desperate attachment to unavailable people: Unconsciously, you might choose people who can't fully commit, recreating the familiar pattern of longing for someone just out of reach. Available people might feel "wrong" or trigger more anxiety than unavailable ones.

The abandonment fear in quiet BPD is often rooted in early attachment trauma. But here's where it gets complex with neurodivergence: being autistic or ADHD in a neurotypical family can create attachment trauma even with well-meaning parents. Your emotional needs weren't met not from malice but from misunderstanding. Your way of connecting wasn't recognized as connection.

Self-Harm as Emotional Regulation: The Hidden Epidemic

Self-harm in quiet BPD often goes unnoticed because it's not always dramatic or visible. It might be:

- Scratching that looks like nervousness

- "Accidents" that happen too often

- Restricting food or binge eating

- Compulsive exercising to the point of injury

- Deliberately triggering your own trauma

- Seeking out situations where you'll be hurt

- Denying yourself basic needs

- Mental self-harm through vicious internal criticism

The function of self-harm in quiet BPD is complex. It might:

- Make internal pain visible and "real"

- Provide sense of control when emotions feel chaotic

- Punish yourself for having needs or feelings

- Create physical pain that's easier to understand than emotional pain

- Bring you back to your body when dissociating

- Release emotional pressure that has no other outlet

- Communicate distress you can't verbalize

When you add autism and ADHD to the mix, self-harm might also be:

- A stim that went too far

- Sensory seeking that becomes harmful

- Response to sensory overload

- Consequence of poor interoception (not noticing damage)

- Impulsive response to emotional overwhelm

- Routine that becomes compulsive

Understanding the multiple functions helps find alternatives that serve the same purpose without damage.

The Trauma-BPD Connection: Chicken or Egg?

Research shows BPD has 46% heritability, with siblings having 4.7 times higher risk. So there's clearly a genetic component. But BPD also strongly correlates with trauma. What's going on?

The answer might be that genetic neurodivergent traits create vulnerability to developing BPD in traumatic environments. If you're born with:

- High emotional sensitivity (could be autism, ADHD, or BPD traits)

- Different sensory processing (autism)

- Executive dysfunction (ADHD)

- Rejection sensitivity (ADHD)

And then experience:

- Misattunement from caregivers who don't understand your needs

- Punishment for natural behaviors

- Social rejection and bullying

- Constant invalidation of your experience

- Lack of appropriate support

The result might be BPD developing as a survival strategy in a hostile environment. Your brain learns that relationships are dangerous but necessary, that you must become what others need, that your true self is unacceptable.

This isn't saying BPD is "just trauma" or "just neurodivergence." It's recognizing that BPD might be what happens when a sensitive nervous system develops in an invalidating environment. The genetic vulnerability meets environmental triggers, creating the perfect storm.

Why Autistic Women Get Misdiagnosed with BPD

The misdiagnosis of autistic women as BPD is so common it's almost predictable. Here's why it happens:

Symptom overlap creates confusion:

- Social difficulties (autism) look like relationship instability (BPD)

- Meltdowns (autism) look like emotional dysregulation (BPD)

- Masking (autism) looks like identity disturbance (BPD)

- Sensory overload (autism) looks like dramatic reactions (BPD)

- Need for sameness (autism) looks like fear of abandonment (BPD)

Gender bias affects interpretation:

- Women's distress gets labeled emotional/relational rather than neurological

- Autism stereotypes miss female presentations
- BPD diagnosis carries less stigma for clinicians than "missed autism"
- Women's self-advocacy gets pathologized as attention-seeking

Masking hides autism:

- By adulthood, autistic women often mask so well that autism isn't considered
- The exhaustion from masking looks like depression
- The identity confusion from masking looks like BPD
- Social scripts look like manipulation rather than communication strategy

Trauma complicates the picture:

- Autistic women experience high rates of trauma
- Trauma responses overlap with both autism and BPD
- Clinicians might stop at trauma/BPD without looking deeper

The tragedy is that misdiagnosis leads to inappropriate treatment. DBT might help with emotional regulation but miss sensory needs. Therapy focused on abandonment won't address social communication differences. Medications for mood might worsen sensory issues.

Building Accurate Self-Understanding

If you're trying to figure out whether you have quiet BPD, autism, ADHD, or all three, here are some differentiating questions:

About emotions:

- Do they feel like yours or like invasions? (BPD: invasions, Autism/ADHD: yours but overwhelming)

- Can you identify them? (Autism: often no, BPD: too many at once, ADHD: after they pass)
- Do they change with people present? (BPD: yes, Autism: maybe, ADHD: less so)

About identity:

- Is there a "you" under the masks? (Autism: yes but hidden, BPD: uncertain, ADHD: yes but inconsistent)
- Do you know what you like when alone? (Autism: yes, BPD: maybe not, ADHD: varies with dopamine)
- Does identity feel empty or just hidden? (BPD: empty, Autism: hidden, ADHD: scattered)

About relationships:

- Do you want them? (Usually yes for all, but differently)
- What's the fear? (BPD: abandonment, Autism: misunderstanding, ADHD: rejection)
- Can you be alone? (BPD: painful, Autism: necessary, ADHD: boring)

About self-harm:

- What triggers it? (BPD: emotional pain, Autism: overload, ADHD: impulse)
- What does it accomplish? (BPD: regulation/punishment, Autism: stimulation/grounding, ADHD: stimulation/focus)
- Is it planned or impulsive? (BPD: both, Autism: might be routine, ADHD: usually impulsive)

Living with Quiet BPD in a Loud World

If quiet BPD is part of your experience, know this: your pain is real even if others can't see it. Your struggles are valid even if you hide them perfectly. You deserve support even if you've learned to never ask for it.

Living with quiet BPD might mean:

- Learning to recognize early warning signs before you implode

- Finding safe ways to express the emotions you've learned to hide

- Building identity through exploration rather than fusion with others

- Developing distress tolerance that doesn't involve self-punishment

- Creating relationships that can hold your intensity without consuming you

- Accepting that healing isn't becoming "normal" but finding sustainable ways to be yourself

The interaction with autism and ADHD means your strategies need to account for all three:

- Emotional regulation that considers sensory needs

- Identity work that accepts neurodivergent authenticity

- Relationship patterns that honor your need for both connection and autonomy

- Treatment approaches that don't pathologize your neurodivergence while addressing genuine suffering

Identity Coherence Assessment

Rate each statement from 1 (never) to 5 (always):

Sense of Self:

- I know who I am when I'm alone

- My values stay consistent regardless of who I'm with

- I can describe myself without referring to others

- My interests remain stable over time

- I feel like the same person in different situations

In Relationships:

- I maintain my opinions even if others disagree

- I can be myself with others

- I know where I end and others begin

- I can tolerate others' disapproval

- My self-worth exists independent of others

Emotional Experience:

- I can identify my emotions

- My emotions feel like they belong to me

- I can predict my emotional patterns

- Emotions pass through me rather than becoming me

- I can self-soothe without self-harm

Look at your patterns. Low scores might indicate BPD identity disturbance, but could also reflect masking, trauma, or neurodivergent identity development.

The Path Forward with Quiet BPD

Recovery from quiet BPD doesn't mean eliminating emotional intensity or becoming someone you're not. It means learning to:

- Direct compassion inward instead of just outward

- Express needs before they become crises

- Build identity that isn't dependent on others

- Tolerate abandonment fears without self-abandonment

- Find safe ways to be seen in your pain

When combined with autism and ADHD, recovery also means:

- Distinguishing between BPD emptiness and autistic burnout

- Recognizing when emotional dysregulation has multiple sources

- Building supports that address all conditions

- Accepting that progress might look different from typical BPD recovery

- Finding clinicians who understand the full picture

The quiet BPD part of you developed for good reasons. It protected you when expressing distress was dangerous. It helped you survive environments that couldn't hold your intensity. Honoring that survival while building new strategies is the path forward.

Your quiet suffering deserves to be heard. Your hidden pain deserves witness. Your internal storm deserves calm. Not through silencing it, but through finding safe ways to let it exist without destroying you.

Armed with this understanding of how quiet BPD interacts with autism and ADHD, you're ready to build practical strategies for emotional regulation that honor all aspects of your neurodivergence.

Chapter 8: The Perfect Storm

When All Three Conditions Overlap

There's a moment when everything clicks. Not in a good way, necessarily. More like when you finally understand why your life has felt like trying to solve three different jigsaw puzzles simultaneously while someone keeps switching the pieces around. ADHD, autism, and BPD traits aren't just coexisting in your brain – they're having a full-on conversation, sometimes in harmony, often in conflict, creating a neurological experience that's uniquely yours and uniquely challenging.

The research tells us these overlaps aren't rare. Genetic correlations between ADHD and autism range from 0.50 to 0.72 – that's massive overlap in genetic architecture. But statistics don't capture what it feels like to live at this intersection, where each condition amplifies and modifies the others in ways that no single diagnosis can explain.

Triple Comorbidity: More Than the Sum of Its Parts

When ADHD, autism, and BPD traits converge, they don't just add up – they multiply, interact, and create entirely new patterns. Think of it like mixing primary colors. Red plus blue gives you purple, but purple isn't just "red and blue" – it's something entirely new with its own properties.

Here's how these conditions typically interact:

ADHD provides the chaos engine – the restlessness, impulsivity, and executive dysfunction that keeps everything in motion. Your brain is always seeking, always moving, never quite settling.

Autism provides the rigidity framework – the need for sameness, the sensory sensitivities, the social confusion that makes the world feel unpredictable and overwhelming.

BPD provides the emotional amplifier – the intensity, the fear of abandonment, the identity confusion that makes every interaction feel like a potential crisis.

Now watch what happens when they interact:

Your ADHD impulsivity clashes with your autistic need for routine, creating a constant internal war between novelty-seeking and sameness-needing. Your BPD emotional dysregulation gets triggered by autistic sensory overload. Your autistic communication differences get interpreted through BPD's abandonment filter, making every social misunderstanding feel like rejection. Your ADHD time blindness prevents you from maintaining the routines that keep your autism regulated. Your BPD identity confusion gets worse because you're constantly masking both ADHD and autism. And round and round it goes.

The Amplification Effect: When Conditions Make Each Other Worse

Each condition doesn't just exist alongside the others – they actively make each other more difficult to manage. This amplification effect is why standard treatments often fail. You're not dealing with three separate issues; you're dealing with an integrated system where touching one part affects everything else.

Consider emotional regulation. ADHD gives you quick-trigger emotions. Autism makes it hard to identify and process those emotions. BPD makes those emotions feel overwhelming and permanent. The combination? Emotional storms that come from nowhere, make no sense, and feel impossible to escape.

Or look at relationships. ADHD makes you forgetful and inconsistent. Autism makes you miss social cues. BPD makes you terrified of abandonment. Together? You desperately want connection but consistently mess it up in ways you don't understand, reinforcing the belief that you're fundamentally unlovable.

Executive function becomes almost impossible. ADHD scatters your attention. Autism demands specific conditions to function. BPD floods you with emotions that shut down your prefrontal cortex. Result? You can't start tasks, can't switch tasks, can't complete tasks, and hate yourself for it.

Trauma: The Fourth Element Nobody Talks About

Here's what complicates everything further: if you have this triple overlap, you almost certainly have trauma. Not necessarily big-T trauma (though that's common too), but the cumulative developmental trauma of being profoundly misunderstood your entire life.

Growing up with undiagnosed or misunderstood neurodivergence is inherently traumatic. You're punished for things you can't control. You're told you're lazy, difficult, too sensitive, not trying hard enough. You fail at things that seem easy for others. You're rejected, bullied, excluded. Your nervous system develops in a state of chronic stress.

This trauma doesn't just sit alongside your neurodivergence – it interweaves with it. Your autistic sensory sensitivities become hypervigilance. Your ADHD emotional dysregulation becomes trauma responses. Your BPD symptoms might partially be how trauma manifests in a neurodivergent nervous system.

Research shows autistic adults have PTSD rates of 32-45% compared to 4-4.5% in the general population. That's not coincidence – it's the predictable result of living in a world not designed for your brain. Add ADHD and BPD traits, and the trauma accumulates exponentially.

Developmental Trajectories: How Did We Get Here?

Understanding how these conditions develop and interact over time helps make sense of your current situation. They don't all appear at once – they unfold in patterns that create cascading effects.

Often, it starts with early neurodivergent traits that go unrecognized. Maybe you were a "sensitive" child (autistic sensory differences), "hyperactive" or "daydreamy" (ADHD), and "intense" (emotional dysregulation). These aren't seen as neurological differences but as personality quirks or behavioral problems.

As you grow, the demands increase. School requires executive function you don't have. Social situations require skills that don't come naturally. You start masking, copying others, working ten times harder than your peers just to appear normal. This exhausting performance becomes your survival strategy.

By adolescence, the cumulative stress starts showing. Anxiety, depression, eating disorders, self-harm – these aren't separate issues but symptoms of a neurodivergent person trying to survive in a neurotypical world. The BPD traits might emerge here, as your overtaxed nervous system and identity confusion from years of masking create emotional instability and relationship chaos.

Adulthood brings new challenges. Work, relationships, independent living – all require executive function and emotional regulation you're struggling to maintain. Burnout becomes cyclical. Mental health crises accumulate. You might get diagnosed with various conditions, try different treatments, but nothing quite fits because nobody's looking at the whole picture.

Gender Diversity and Neurodivergence: The Intersection Within Intersections

Here's a statistical reality that changes everything: gender-diverse individuals are 3-6 times more likely to be autistic, with similar elevations in ADHD rates. This isn't coincidence – there's something fundamental about how neurodivergence and gender diversity intersect.

Maybe it's that neurodivergent brains are less constrained by social categories. Maybe it's that the experience of being neurodivergent – of never quite fitting in – creates space to question other social norms like gender. Maybe it's that the same genetic or neurological factors influence both neurodevelopment and gender identity.

For many people with this triple overlap, gender identity becomes another layer of complexity. You're not just managing ADHD, autism, and BPD traits – you're also navigating gender dysphoria, social transition, medical transition, or simply existing outside the gender binary in a world that demands you pick a box.

This intersection creates unique challenges:

- Medical gatekeeping that pathologizes both neurodivergence and gender diversity

- Having to mask multiple aspects of identity simultaneously

- Difficulty accessing appropriate care that understands all aspects

- Increased minority stress from multiple marginalized identities

- But also: finding community with others who exist at similar intersections

Creating Your Personal Condition Map

Understanding your unique presentation means mapping how these conditions show up specifically in your life. Not how they appear in textbooks, but how they manifest in your daily experience.

Start with the overlaps. Where do symptoms blur together? Which traits belong to which condition, and does it even matter? Sometimes trying to separate them is less useful than understanding how they interact.

Map your triggers and cascades. What sets off chains of symptoms? How does sensory overload (autism) lead to emotional dysregulation (BPD) which depletes executive function (ADHD)? Understanding these patterns helps you intervene earlier in the cascade.

Identify your masking strategies. How do you hide each condition? What energy does it take? Where has masking become so automatic you don't even notice it anymore? This awareness is the first step to reducing masking's toll.

Notice your regulation strategies. What actually helps? Not what should help according to experts, but what works for your specific brain. Maybe it's stimming while doing ADHD body doubling during a specific time of day when your BPD symptoms are quietest. Your strategies might seem weird to others but make perfect sense for your neurological profile.

The Professional Challenge: Finding Help That Gets It

Here's a hard truth: most professionals aren't equipped to understand this level of complexity. They're trained to look for and treat single conditions. When you present with this triple overlap plus trauma plus possibly gender diversity, you overwhelm the system.

You might encounter:

- Professionals who insist you can't have all three conditions

- Treatments that help one condition while worsening others

- Medication trials that produce unexpected results

- Therapy that doesn't account for neurodivergence

- Dismissal of your experience as "too complex"

Finding appropriate help often means:

- Seeking specialists who understand neurodevelopmental conditions in adults

- Building a team rather than relying on one provider

- Educating your providers about your specific presentation

- Being willing to try unconventional approaches

- Accepting that you might know more about your conditions than some professionals

Living at the Intersection: Daily Reality

What does daily life actually look like with this triple overlap? It might mean:

Mornings where you need your ADHD medication to function but it increases your autistic sensory sensitivity and your BPD emotional volatility. Choosing which symptoms to manage and which to endure.

Work days where you're masking autism in meetings, managing ADHD symptoms with extensive systems, and controlling BPD emotions through sheer will, then coming home and completely collapsing.

Relationships where you're simultaneously desperate for connection (BPD), overwhelmed by social interaction (autism), and inconsistent in maintaining contact (ADHD). Partners who don't understand why you're intensely present one day and completely withdrawn the next.

A constant juggling act of competing needs. Your autism needs routine but your ADHD needs novelty. Your BPD needs reassurance but your autism needs space. Your ADHD needs stimulation but your autism needs calm. There's no perfect solution, only constant negotiation.

Building a Life That Works

Living with this complex presentation isn't about fixing yourself or making the symptoms go away. It's about building a life that accommodates your neurological reality. This might mean:

Radical acceptance of your limitations. You might never be able to work full-time in an office. You might need more support than others your age. That's not failure; it's reality.

Creative solutions that work for your specific brain. Maybe you work from home at weird hours. Maybe you communicate primarily through text. Maybe your relationships look different from the norm. If it works for you, it's valid.

Layers of support systems. Not relying on one person or strategy but building redundant supports. Multiple coping strategies, various support people, different professional resources.

Flexible structure. Enough routine to keep your autism regulated but enough flexibility for ADHD needs and BPD emotional variability. Structure that bends without breaking.

Energy management as priority. Recognizing that you're using enormous energy just to exist and planning accordingly. This might mean saying no to most things to preserve energy for what matters.

Community with others at similar intersections. Finding your people – other multiply neurodivergent folks who get it without explanation. Online spaces can be lifelines when in-person community is inaccessible.

The Integration Path: Making Peace with Complexity

Living at this intersection means accepting that your experience will always be complex. You're not going to wake up one day with a simple, straightforward neurology. But complexity doesn't mean chaos. Understanding how your conditions interact gives you power to work with your brain rather than against it.

Integration doesn't mean the conditions merge into one thing. It means understanding how they dance together in your specific nervous system. It means recognizing patterns, predicting cascades, and building strategies that account for all aspects of your neurology.

Some days, one condition will dominate. Other days, they'll all be quiet. Some days, they'll all be screaming at once. This variability is part of your pattern, not evidence of failure or faking.

Personal Condition Mapping Exercise

Create your own intersection map:

1. **Draw three overlapping circles** for ADHD, autism, and BPD traits

2. **In each individual circle**, list symptoms unique to that condition

3. **In the overlaps**, note symptoms that could belong to multiple conditions

4. **In the center where all three meet**, identify your most complex symptoms

5. **Around the outside**, add trauma responses and coping mechanisms

Look at your map. This is your neurological landscape. It's complex, but it's yours, and understanding it is the first step to navigating it.

With this scaffolding erected for understanding your complex neurology, let's explore how trauma and masking have shaped your identity and how to find yourself beneath all the layers.

Chapter 9: Trauma, Masking, and Identity

The Hidden Factors

Here's something nobody tells you about being multiply neurodivergent: by the time you figure out who you are, you've often forgotten who you were. Years or decades of masking, adapting, and surviving have created so many layers between you and your authentic self that finding your way back feels impossible. Add trauma to the mix – which, let's be honest, is basically inevitable when you're this neurologically complex – and the question "who am I?" becomes almost unanswerable.

But here's the thing: that authentic self isn't gone. It's buried, maybe, compressed under years of performance and pain, but it's still there. The journey to find it might be the hardest thing you ever do, but it's also the most necessary.

Developmental Trauma vs. Neurodivergence: Untangling the Threads

One of the most confusing aspects of being multiply neurodivergent is figuring out what's trauma and what's neurology. They're so intertwined that separating them might be impossible – and maybe that's okay. Maybe the distinction matters less than understanding how they interact.

Developmental trauma happens when a child's emotional and psychological needs aren't met consistently. For neurodivergent kids, this is almost universal. Not because parents are cruel (though sometimes they are), but because the world isn't set up for neurodivergent needs. Your sensory needs weren't understood. Your communication style wasn't recognized. Your emotional intensity was "too much."

This creates a specific type of trauma:

- **Attachment trauma** from caregivers who couldn't attune to your needs

- **Social trauma** from peer rejection and bullying

- **Educational trauma** from school systems that punished your differences

- **Medical trauma** from professionals who pathologized your traits

- **Identity trauma** from being told you're wrong for existing as you are

But here's where it gets complex: trauma symptoms and neurodivergent traits overlap significantly. Sensory sensitivity could be autism or hypervigilance from trauma. Emotional dysregulation could be ADHD, BPD, or trauma responses. Social difficulties could be autistic communication differences or trauma-based withdrawal.

The truth? It's probably both. Your neurodivergence made you more vulnerable to trauma, and trauma shaped how your neurodivergence manifests. They're not separate threads but a woven fabric of your experience.

The Masking Machine: How We Learned to Disappear

Masking didn't start as a choice. It started as survival. Maybe you were three years old, noticing that flapping your hands made adults uncomfortable. Maybe you were seven, realizing that talking about your special interest made other kids roll their eyes. Maybe you were twelve, discovering that pretending to be someone else made you less of a target.

Each small adjustment seemed reasonable at the time. Stop stimming. Make eye contact. Laugh when others laugh. Say what people want to hear. Follow social scripts even when they make no sense. Hide your struggles. Pretend everything's fine.

But masking isn't just behavioral – it's neurological. Your brain literally rewires itself to maintain the performance. Neural pathways strengthen for monitoring and mimicry while pathways for self-expression atrophy. You become an expert at being whoever others need you to be, but you lose track of who you are.

The cost accumulates:

- **Cognitive overload** from constant monitoring and adjustment

- **Emotional exhaustion** from suppressing your natural responses

- **Identity confusion** from playing so many roles

- **Physical symptoms** from chronic stress

- **Mental health crises** when the mask cracks

- **Autistic burnout** when masking becomes impossible

Research shows that camouflaging autistic traits is associated with increased depression, anxiety, and suicidality. The same patterns exist for ADHD and BPD masking. When you're masking all three conditions, the toll is exponential.

Identity Diffusion: Who Am I Under All These Masks?

Identity formation is already complex for neurodivergent people. Add years of masking and trauma, and identity becomes a maze with no exit. You might experience:

The chameleon effect: You unconsciously mirror whoever you're with, taking on their interests, mannerisms, even opinions. You're a different person with different people, and none of them feel real.

The imposter syndrome: Even when you succeed, it feels fake because you achieved it while masking. You're constantly afraid of being "found out," though you're not sure what there is to find.

The empty core: When you're alone, you feel hollow. Without someone to mirror or a role to play, you don't know who you are or what you want. The silence is deafening.

The fragment collection: You feel like pieces of different people rather than a whole person. Each fragment makes sense in context but they don't form a coherent whole.

This isn't a character flaw or psychological weakness. It's the predictable result of never being safe to be yourself. Your identity went underground to survive, and now you need to coax it back out.

The Mental Health Cost of Camouflaging

The statistics are sobering. Autistic adults who mask more show higher rates of depression, anxiety, and suicidal ideation. People with ADHD who hide their symptoms develop anxiety disorders at higher rates. Those with BPD who suppress their emotional intensity often develop severe depression.

But statistics don't capture the lived experience:

The bone-deep exhaustion that sleep doesn't fix. The anxiety that pervades everything because you're constantly performing. The depression that comes from living an inauthentic life. The dissociation from being disconnected from yourself. The rage that builds from suppressing your needs. The grief for the person you might have been.

Mental health treatment often fails because it doesn't address the root cause. Treating depression without addressing masking is like bailing water from a boat without patching the hole. The symptoms might temporarily improve, but the underlying dynamic remains.

Neurodivergent Trauma: The Wounds Nobody Sees

Beyond developmental trauma, neurodivergent people experience specific types of trauma that neurotypical people rarely encounter:

Sensory trauma: Being forced to endure sensory experiences that are genuinely painful. Fluorescent lights that feel like assault. Textures that make you want to claw your skin off. Sounds that scramble your thoughts. Years of being told you're "too sensitive" when you're in actual pain.

Social trauma: Not just rejection but complete bewilderment. Watching others navigate social situations effortlessly while you struggle with every interaction. Being punished for social mistakes you didn't know you were making. The accumulated wound of a thousand microaggressions.

Communication trauma: Having your communication style consistently invalidated. Being told you're too direct, too intense, too much, not enough. Having your words twisted, your intentions misunderstood, your needs dismissed. Learning that your natural way of connecting is wrong.

Identity trauma: Being pathologized for existing. Having your traits labeled as disorders. Being told you need to be fixed. Internalizing the message that there's something fundamentally wrong with you.

Systemic trauma: Fighting systems that don't accommodate you. Schools that punish your needs. Workplaces that demand masking. Healthcare that doesn't understand you. Support systems that require you to be sicker to get help but not so sick that you're "non-compliant."

Breaking Intergenerational Cycles

Here's something that might blow your mind: your neurodivergence likely runs in your family, which means trauma patterns do too. Your parents might be undiagnosed neurodivergent people who learned to mask and passed those survival strategies to you.

Think about it. That anxious parent who needed everything perfect? Might have been masking ADHD chaos. That emotionally distant parent? Might have been autistic and overwhelmed. That parent with

78

intense, unpredictable emotions? Might have been dealing with their own BPD traits.

This isn't about blame. They were doing their best with brains that nobody understood in a world that was even less accommodating than today. But recognizing these patterns helps you understand:

- Why certain family dynamics feel so familiar yet so wrong

- How trauma responses get passed down as "normal" behavior

- Why getting healthier might feel like betraying family patterns

- How breaking cycles means grieving what multiple generations lost

Breaking these cycles doesn't mean cutting off family (unless that's what you need). It means recognizing patterns, understanding their origins, and consciously choosing different responses. It means being the generation that says, "This stops with me."

Building Authentic Identity After Years of Masking

Finding yourself after decades of masking isn't a quick process. It's archaeology – carefully excavating layers, examining what you find, deciding what to keep. Here's what this might look like:

Start with the body: Your body remembers who you are even when your mind forgets. What movements feel good? What sensory experiences bring relief? What makes your nervous system settle? Your authentic self often speaks through sensation before words.

Notice micro-moments of authenticity: When do you feel most yourself? Maybe it's alone at 3 AM. Maybe it's with your pet. Maybe it's doing your special interest. These moments are breadcrumbs leading back to yourself.

Experiment with unmasking: Start small and safe. Stim in private. Say no to something you'd usually force yourself through. Express an opinion without softening it. Notice what happens – both the relief and the fear.

Grieve who you could have been: This is brutal but necessary. Grieve the life you might have had if you'd been diagnosed earlier, supported better, understood more. Grieve the energy spent masking. Grieve the connections lost to misunderstanding. Let yourself feel the magnitude of the loss.

Explore without attachment: Try things without committing to them being "you." Experiment with presentation, interests, communication styles. You're not building a new mask but discovering what fits when you're not trying to fit.

Connect with other unmasking people: Find communities of people on similar journeys. Seeing others reclaim authenticity gives you permission to do the same. Their courage becomes your courage.

The Window of Tolerance in Neurodivergent Nervous Systems

The "window of tolerance" concept needs major modification for neurodivergent folks. The traditional model assumes a stable baseline, but your baseline might shift hourly based on:

- Sensory accumulation
- Social battery depletion
- Executive function availability
- Emotional regulation capacity
- Masking fatigue
- Trauma activation

Your window might be narrow in some areas (sensory tolerance) but wide in others (crisis management). It might be different at different times of day, month, or year. Understanding your unique window helps you:

- Recognize when you're approaching edges
- Develop strategies for different zones
- Communicate your needs before crisis
- Build routines that keep you regulated
- Accept your variability without judgment

The Path Forward: Integration Not Elimination

Healing from trauma and reducing masking doesn't mean your neurodivergence goes away. You're not trying to become neurotypical – that's neither possible nor desirable. You're learning to be authentically neurodivergent in a world that's slowly (very slowly) becoming more accommodating.

Integration means:

- Acknowledging all parts of your experience
- Understanding how trauma and neurodivergence interact
- Developing strategies that work for your specific brain
- Building relationships that don't require masking
- Creating environments that support your needs
- Accepting that healing is nonlinear

Some days you'll mask because it's safer. Some days trauma will overwhelm your coping strategies. Some days you'll feel like you're back at square one. This isn't failure – it's the reality of living with complex neurology in a complex world.

Creating Your Unmasking Timeline

This isn't about forcing yourself to unmask before you're ready. It's about consciously choosing when, where, and how much to reveal. Consider:

Safe spaces first: Where can you practice being authentic with minimal risk?

Gradual revelation: What small aspects of yourself can you stop hiding?

Support systems: Who can support you as you unmask?

Backup plans: What will you do if unmasking goes poorly?

Energy management: How will you handle the initial increase in energy from not masking?

Identity anchors: What reminds you who you are when you feel lost?

The Truth About Finding Yourself

Here's what I've learned from watching hundreds of people navigate this journey: finding yourself after trauma and masking isn't a destination. It's an ongoing process of becoming. You don't find a fixed "true self" underneath the masks – you discover that you're allowed to be fluid, complex, contradictory.

Your authentic self might be:

- Different in different contexts (and that's okay)

- Constantly evolving (and that's okay)

- Sometimes unclear even to you (and that's okay)

- Messier than any diagnosis can capture (and that's okay)

The goal isn't to become a fixed, stable person. It's to develop enough self-knowledge and self-acceptance that you can navigate your complexity with compassion instead of criticism, curiosity instead of judgment.

Identity Archaeology Exercise

Take some time to excavate your authentic self:

1. **Before the masks** (ages 0-5): What do you remember about your earliest self? What brought you joy? What felt natural?

2. **The first masks** (ages 6-12): When did you first realize you were different? What did you start hiding? What strategies did you develop?

3. **The performance** (adolescence): How did masking intensify? What roles did you play? What was the cost?

4. **The cracks** (when things started breaking down): When did masking stop working? What crises emerged? What forced you to reconsider?

5. **The revelation** (discovering neurodivergence): How did understanding your neurology change things? What made sense in retrospect?

6. **The integration** (now): What parts of yourself are you reclaiming? What masks are you keeping by choice? Who are you becoming?

Look at this timeline with compassion. Every adaptation was survival. Every mask was protection. Now you get to choose what serves you and what you're ready to release.

Having cleared this conceptual space around trauma and identity, you're ready to build practical strategies for living with your unique neurology.

Chapter 10: The Neurodivergent DBT Toolkit

Emotional Regulation Strategies

Traditional DBT assumes a neurotypical brain. It assumes you can identify emotions, tolerate distress without sensory overload, and communicate needs in neurotypical ways. When you're dealing with ADHD, autism, and BPD traits simultaneously, standard DBT needs serious modification. Not because the core concepts are wrong, but because they need translation into neurodivergent language and adaptation for different neurological wiring.

What works isn't abandoning DBT but rebuilding it from the ground up with neurodivergent needs centered. This means accounting for alexithymia, sensory processing differences, executive dysfunction, and communication styles that don't fit the neurotypical mold. It means recognizing that your distress might be sensory, your emotions might be delayed, and your interpersonal effectiveness might look completely different from the textbook examples.

Distress Tolerance When Your Nervous System Works Differently

The classic TIPP skills (Temperature, Intense exercise, Paced breathing, Paired muscle relaxation) need major adjustments for neurodivergent nervous systems. Your sensory profile, executive function, and emotional processing all affect what actually helps versus what makes things worse.

Temperature works differently when you have sensory processing differences. Cold water on your face might be overwhelming rather than grounding. Ice might cause sensory shock that increases distress. Instead, you might need:

- Weighted blankets for deep pressure

- Warm baths with specific textures (bubbles, salts)

- Temperature changes you control (holding ice wrapped in fabric)

- Alternating temperatures rather than sudden changes

Intense exercise gets complicated with motor planning difficulties, sensory sensitivities, and executive dysfunction. Running might be impossible when you're dysregulated, but stimming is movement too. Try:

- Vigorous stimming (jumping, rocking, flapping)

- Isometric exercises that don't require coordination

- Sensory-based movement (spinning, swinging)

- Repetitive movements that don't require planning

Paced breathing assumes you can feel your breath and control it consciously. With poor interoception or anxiety about breathing, this might increase panic. Alternatives include:

- Visual breathing guides (watching shapes expand/contract)

- Counting without breath focus

- Humming or singing for breath regulation

- Movement-based breathing (arms up on inhale, down on exhale)

Paired muscle relaxation requires body awareness many neurodivergent people lack. Plus, the sensation might be uncomfortable. Consider:

- Compression clothing for consistent pressure

- Self-squeezing or self-hugging

- Using tools (stress balls, therapy putty)

- Progressive pressure rather than tension-release

The key is finding what regulates YOUR specific nervous system, not following a formula that assumes neurotypical sensory processing.

Emotional Regulation When You Can't Name Emotions

Alexithymia – difficulty identifying and describing emotions – affects up to 50% of autistic people and is common in ADHD and BPD too. Standard emotion regulation assumes you know what you're feeling. But what if emotions are just "bad," "weird," or "something"?

Start with body sensations rather than emotion labels:

- Where do you feel it? (chest, stomach, head, limbs)

- What's the quality? (tight, hot, buzzy, heavy, empty)

- Is it moving or still? (spreading, pulsing, stuck)

- What does it want to do? (run, hide, fight, collapse)

Build your personal emotion-sensation dictionary:

- Anger might be heat in chest plus clenched jaw

- Anxiety might be stomach butterflies plus racing thoughts

- Sadness might be heaviness plus slow thoughts

- Joy might be chest lightness plus energy in limbs

Use contexts and triggers as clues:

- What just happened?

- What thoughts are present?

- What urges do you have?

- What would help right now?

Sometimes you won't know what emotion it is, and that's okay. You can still regulate "the uncomfortable thing in my chest" without naming it anxiety.

Interpersonal Effectiveness for Different Communication Styles

DBT's interpersonal effectiveness assumes neurotypical communication – subtle cues, indirect requests, reading between lines. For neurodivergent folks, we need different scripts that account for:

- Direct communication preferences
- Difficulty with nonverbal cues
- Processing delays
- Sensory factors affecting interaction
- Different relationship needs

DEAR MAN (Describe, Express, Assert, Reinforce, Mindful, Appear confident, Negotiate) becomes:

Describe with concrete specifics, not hints:

- "You said you'd call at 3 PM and didn't" not "You forgot about me"
- Include sensory/practical impacts: "The uncertainty makes my chest tight"

Express using sensation/need language if emotions are unclear:

- "I need predictability" rather than "I feel anxious"
- "My body is activated" rather than trying to name complex emotions

Assert with clear, direct requests:

- No hints, implications, or hoping they'll figure it out
- "I need you to text if plans change" not "It would be nice if..."

Reinforce by explaining YOUR brain's needs:

- "This helps my autism brain feel safe"
- "My ADHD needs this structure to function"

Mindful means managing YOUR sensory/emotional state:

- Take breaks if overwhelmed
- Stim if needed
- Use written communication if verbal is too hard

Appear confident doesn't mean masking:

- Confidence can include stating your needs matter
- You can be confident while stimming or avoiding eye contact

Negotiate with your limitations acknowledged:

- "I can do X if you can do Y"
- "This is a need, not a preference"

Mindfulness for Busy, Scattered, Sensory Brains

Traditional mindfulness meditation might be torture for ADHD brains, overwhelming for autistic sensory systems, or triggering for trauma survivors. But mindfulness isn't just sitting still and breathing. It's present-moment awareness, which can happen many ways.

Movement-based mindfulness:

- Walking meditation with counting steps

- Stimming with full attention
- Dance or rhythmic movement
- Stretching with body awareness

Sensory mindfulness:

- Focus on one pleasant sensory input
- Mindful stimming (really feeling the sensation)
- Temperature awareness
- Texture exploration

Special interest mindfulness:

- Deep engagement with your interest
- Hyperfocus as meditation
- Info-dumping as present-moment joy
- Creating/organizing within your interest

ADHD-friendly mindfulness:

- Very short sessions (30 seconds is enough)
- Fidget-friendly meditation
- Background music or white noise
- Multiple short sessions vs. one long one

Autism-friendly mindfulness:

- Predictable structure
- Same time, place, position
- Visual or tactile anchors
- Avoiding overwhelming sensory input

The goal isn't to achieve some mythical calm state but to be present with whatever IS, including restlessness, sensory input, and busy thoughts.

Crisis Planning That Accounts for Neurodivergent Needs

Standard crisis plans assume you can communicate verbally, access resources independently, and implement coping strategies without support. Neurodivergent crisis planning needs to account for:

Communication differences:

- Pre-written texts to send when nonverbal

- Code words for different crisis types

- Visual cards showing needs

- Designated person who understands your communication style

Sensory needs:

- Specific sensory tools ready (weighted blanket, noise-canceling headphones, safe foods)

- Environmental modifications (dimmed lights, quiet space)

- Sensory first-aid kit portable and accessible

Executive dysfunction:

- Step-by-step crisis protocol written out

- Visual guides for coping strategies

- Pre-packed crisis bag

- Automated reminders for basic needs

Support needs:

- Clear instructions for support people

- What helps vs. what makes things worse

- How to tell if you need professional help

- Backup plans if primary support unavailable

Your crisis plan should assume you'll have minimal capacity and maximum need. Everything should be as simple, clear, and accessible as possible.

Building Your Personal DBT Adaptation

Standard DBT modules need personalization for your specific neurodivergent profile. This means identifying:

Which skills actually work for your brain:

- What genuinely reduces distress?

- What's accessible during dysregulation?

- What fits your sensory profile?

- What works with your executive function?

Your skill hierarchy:

- Tier 1: Always accessible (stimming, compression)

- Tier 2: Usually accessible (breathing, movement)

- Tier 3: Sometimes accessible (complex skills)

- Tier 4: Only when regulated (interpersonal skills)

Your implementation barriers:

- Sensory obstacles

- Executive function challenges

- Communication differences

- Environmental factors

Your support needs:

- When can you self-implement?

- When do you need prompting?

- When do you need active support?

- When do you need professional help?

The Reality of Emotional Regulation with Complex Neurology

Here's what they don't tell you in standard DBT: when you have ADHD, autism, and BPD traits, emotional regulation isn't a skill you master. It's an ongoing negotiation with a nervous system that plays by different rules. Some days, all your skills work. Other days, you can barely access one. This isn't failure – it's the reality of complex neurology.

Progress looks different too. It might mean:

- Shorter recovery time rather than preventing dysregulation

- Recognizing triggers earlier even if you can't avoid them

- Having more tools even if each works only sometimes

- Reducing harm even if you can't eliminate distress

- Communicating needs even if they can't always be met

The goal isn't neurotypical emotional regulation. It's finding what works for YOUR brain, in YOUR life, with YOUR specific combination of traits. That might look nothing like textbook DBT, and that's perfectly fine.

DBT Skills Adaptation Worksheet

For each DBT skill category, identify:

Distress Tolerance:

- Standard skill that doesn't work and why

- Your adaptation that does work

- When it's accessible

- What support you need

Emotion Regulation:

- How you identify emotions

- What helps you regulate

- Your early warning signs

- Your recovery strategies

Interpersonal Effectiveness:

- Your communication style

- Scripts that work for you

- Relationship needs

- Boundary strategies

Mindfulness:

- Types that work for your brain

- Duration you can manage

- Best times/conditions

- Adaptations needed

This becomes your personalized DBT manual, built for your specific neurodivergent needs.

These building blocks enable us to expand into environmental adaptations and sensory strategies that support your daily functioning.

Chapter 11: Sensory Strategies and Environmental Design

Your environment is talking to your nervous system constantly, and if you're multiply neurodivergent, it's usually shouting. That fluorescent light isn't just annoying – it's scrambling your brain. That background noise isn't just distracting – it's depleting your cognitive resources. That scratchy tag isn't just uncomfortable – it's activating your fight-or-flight response. When you have ADHD, autism, and BPD traits, your environment can make the difference between functioning and complete dysregulation.

Most advice about environmental modification assumes you have complete control over your space and unlimited resources to change it. Reality? You're probably dealing with shared spaces, limited budgets, and environments you can't modify. But there are still ways to create pockets of sensory safety, even in hostile sensory environments.

Creating Sensory-Friendly Spaces in an Unfriendly World

Start with understanding that "sensory-friendly" means different things for different parts of your neurodivergent profile. Your ADHD might crave stimulation while your autism needs calm. Your BPD emotional states might change your sensory needs hour by hour. The key is creating flexible spaces that can adapt to your changing needs.

Lighting is often the first sensory assault. Fluorescent lights are basically kryptonite for many neurodivergent people. They flicker at frequencies that might be below conscious awareness but still affect your nervous system. Options include:

- Lamp lighting instead of overhead lights

- Smart bulbs that adjust color temperature

- Fairy lights for gentle ambient lighting

- Natural light when possible (but with window coverings for control)

- Light filters for computer screens

- Sunglasses indoors (yes, it's okay)

Sound is the invisible enemy. You might not consciously notice the refrigerator hum, air conditioner buzz, or neighbor's TV, but your nervous system is processing it all. Sound management includes:

- White noise machines (or apps) to mask unpredictable sounds

- Noise-canceling headphones for overwhelming environments

- Earplugs that reduce volume without blocking everything

- Music that regulates YOUR nervous system (not what "should" be calming)

- Silent zones where no unnecessary noise is allowed

- Communication with others about noise needs

Texture and touch affect everything from clothing to furniture. That slightly wrong texture can derail your entire day. Consider:

- Clothing that feels safe (buy multiples when you find something that works)

- Removing or covering irritating textures

- Adding pleasant textures (soft blankets, smooth stones)

- Furniture that supports your sensory needs

- Tools and objects that feel good to touch

- Permission to avoid textures that distress you

Organization and visual environment matter more than neurotypical people realize. Visual clutter might overwhelm your autistic brain while complete minimalism might understimulate your ADHD. Find balance through:

- Closed storage to reduce visual input
- Designated spaces for everything
- Color coding for quick visual processing
- Clear containers so you don't forget what exists
- Minimizing patterns that create visual noise
- Creating visual rest spaces

Workplace Accommodations That Actually Help

The workplace is often sensory hell. Open offices, fluorescent lights, constant interruptions, social demands – it's designed to be difficult for neurodivergent nervous systems. But you have rights, and accommodations aren't special treatment – they're leveling the playing field.

Potential accommodations include:

Environmental modifications:

- Desk location away from high-traffic areas
- Permission to use lamp lighting
- Noise-canceling headphones permitted
- Private workspace when possible
- Control over immediate environment

Schedule modifications:

- Flexible hours to avoid sensory-heavy commutes

- Work from home options

- Regular breaks for sensory regulation

- Predictable schedule when possible

- Advance notice of changes

Communication accommodations:

- Written communication preferred

- Agenda before meetings

- Permission to turn off camera in video calls

- Email summaries after verbal instructions

- Extra processing time for decisions

Task modifications:

- Breaking large projects into smaller steps

- Written instructions for complex tasks

- Regular check-ins instead of vague deadlines

- Permission to work on single tasks vs. multitasking

- Flexibility in how tasks are completed

The key to getting accommodations is being specific about how they help you perform essential job functions. Not "I don't like fluorescent lights" but "Fluorescent lights trigger sensory overload that impairs my concentration, affecting my ability to complete detailed work."

Managing Sensory Overload in Daily Life

Sensory overload isn't just uncomfortable – it's neurologically overwhelming. Your brain literally cannot process more input, leading to shutdown, meltdown, or dissociation. Managing it means both prevention and recovery strategies.

Prevention through sensory budgeting: Think of sensory tolerance like a budget. Every sensory input spends some. Overwhelming inputs might blow the whole budget at once. This means:

- Planning high-sensory activities when you have capacity
- Building in recovery time after sensory challenges
- Saying no to protect sensory bandwidth
- Creating low-sensory zones in your day
- Using sensory supports proactively, not just reactively

Early warning recognition:

- Physical signs (tension, headache, stomach upset)
- Cognitive signs (difficulty processing, confusion)
- Emotional signs (irritability, anxiety, numbness)
- Behavioral signs (stimming increase, withdrawal)
- Sensory signs (everything too loud/bright/intense)

In-the-moment strategies:

- Remove or reduce input immediately
- Deep pressure (weighted blanket, compression)
- Single sensory focus (one calming input)
- Movement that works for you
- Communicate needs if possible

Recovery protocols:

- Complete sensory rest if possible
- Gradual re-introduction of input
- Gentle, preferred sensory input

- No demands during recovery

- Time – often more than expected

The Sensory Diet Concept (Redesigned for Adult Life)

"Sensory diet" sounds childish, but it's really about intentionally providing your nervous system with the input it needs to regulate. As an adult with ADHD, autism, and BPD traits, your sensory diet might need to include seemingly contradictory elements.

Your sensory diet might include:

Alerting input (for ADHD understimulation):

- Bright lights when needed

- Loud or complex music

- Strong flavors or temperatures

- Vigorous movement

- Novel sensory experiences

Calming input (for autistic overload):

- Deep pressure

- Rhythmic movement

- Predictable sensory input

- Soft textures

- Familiar sensory experiences

Organizing input (for general regulation):

- Bilateral movement

- Rhythm and pattern

- Proprioceptive input (body awareness)

- Vestibular input (balance/movement)

- Oral sensory input (chewing, sucking)

The key is timing and combination. You might need alerting input in the morning, organizing input midday, and calming input in evening. Or you might need all three simultaneously – loud music while under a weighted blanket doing repetitive movement.

Technology Tools and Apps for Sensory Regulation

Technology can be a powerful sensory regulation tool when used intentionally. Your phone might be overstimulating, but it can also provide crucial sensory support.

Helpful apps and tools include:

- Noise generators (white, pink, brown noise)

- Visual stimmers (patterns, colors, movement)

- Breathing guides with visual/audio/haptic cues

- Reminder apps for sensory breaks

- Communication apps for nonverbal times

- Light filter apps for screens

- Sensory tracking apps

- Virtual reality for controlled sensory input

The trick is using technology as a tool, not a trap. Set boundaries, use intentionally, and remember that digital sensory input is still sensory input that can overload your system.

Building Routine While Maintaining Flexibility

Here's the central paradox: your autism craves routine while your ADHD rebels against it, and your BPD means emotional states can derail any structure. The solution isn't rigid routine or complete chaos but flexible structure – routine with escape hatches.

Flexible structure looks like:

- Core routines that are non-negotiable (medication, sleep)
- Flexible routines with options (morning routine with variations)
- Emergency overrides for bad days
- Seasonal adjustments for changing needs
- Regular routine evaluation and modification

Building sustainable routines:

- Start tiny (one element at a time)
- Attach to existing habits
- Make it sensory-pleasant
- Build in rewards/dopamine
- Allow for imperfection
- Have backup plans

When routines break:

- It's not failure, it's information
- What caused the break?
- What need wasn't being met?
- How can you modify rather than abandon?
- What's the minimum viable routine?

Creating Your Sensory Emergency Kit

Every neurodivergent person needs a sensory emergency kit – portable sensory regulation tools for when you're away from your safe spaces. This isn't optional; it's survival equipment.

Your kit might include:

- Noise-reducing earplugs
- Sunglasses
- Favorite safe food
- Fidget tools
- Compression items (scarf that can wrap tight)
- Scent that grounds you
- Smooth stone or fabric
- Phone with regulation apps
- Communication cards
- Comfort object

The key is having it ready and accessible. Keep one in your car, one at work, one in your bag. When you need it, you won't have executive function to assemble it.

The Environmental Activism of Existing

Here's something radical: creating sensory-accessible environments isn't just self-care – it's activism. Every time you advocate for your sensory needs, you're making space for others who can't advocate yet. Every accommodation you receive makes it easier for the next person.

This might mean:

- Being open about sensory needs
- Requesting accommodations even when scared
- Supporting others' sensory needs
- Challenging sensory-hostile design

- Creating sensory-friendly spaces where you can

- Educating others about sensory needs

Your sensory needs are not "preferences" or "being difficult." They're neurological requirements for functioning. The world won't become sensory-friendly overnight, but every small change matters.

Environmental Audit Checklist

For each environment you regularly inhabit:

Sensory Input Assessment:

- Lighting (type, control, alternatives)

- Sound (sources, volume, control)

- Texture (clothing, furniture, unavoidable touches)

- Smell (present, changeable, tolerable)

- Visual (clutter, patterns, rest spaces)

- Movement (space to move, stillness required)

Modification Possibilities:

- What can you change immediately?

- What requires permission/negotiation?

- What requires resources you don't have yet?

- What absolutely cannot change?

Coping Strategies:

- How can you modify your experience?

- What tools help in this space?

- When is this space most/least tolerable?

- How can you limit time or recover after?

This assessment becomes your environmental modification roadmap.

From this vantage point of environmental awareness, we can explore how to build relationships and community that honor your neurodivergent needs.

Chapter 12: Relationships, Communication, and Community

Relationships are hard enough when your brain works one way. When you're juggling ADHD, autism, and BPD traits, relationships become a complex dance where you're simultaneously trying to remember the steps, process the music, and manage your fear that your partner will leave mid-dance. Add in the fact that most relationship advice assumes neurotypical communication styles and emotional processing, and it's no wonder relationships feel impossible.

But here's what I've learned: neurodivergent people can have deeply fulfilling relationships. They just might not look like the neurotypical model. They might require more explicit communication, different intimacy patterns, and creative solutions to common challenges. The key is stop trying to do relationships the "normal" way and start doing them in ways that work for your specific neurology.

Explaining Your Needs Without Apologizing for Existing

One of the hardest parts of being multiply neurodivergent is explaining needs that seem contradictory. How do you explain that you desperately want connection but need to be alone? That you love someone but can't handle physical touch right now? That you're not angry but your face might look like it? That you care deeply but forgot their birthday exists?

Start with education, not justification:

- "My brain processes things differently"

- "I have neurological differences that affect..."

- "This isn't a choice or preference, it's how I'm wired"

- "I care about you, AND I have these needs"

Be specific about what you need:

- Not "I need space" but "I need two hours of alone time to regulate my sensory system"

- Not "I can't handle this" but "I need to process this in writing before we discuss it"

- Not "You're too much" but "I'm at sensory capacity and need to reduce input"

Explain the why when helpful:

- "My autism means I need routine to feel safe"

- "My ADHD makes me forget things that aren't in front of me"

- "My emotional dysregulation means I need time to identify what I'm feeling"

But also: you don't owe anyone endless explanation. Sometimes "this is what I need" is enough. People who care about you will work with that.

Dating While Neurodivergent: The Things Nobody Tells You

Dating with multiple neurodivergent conditions is like playing a video game where the controls keep changing and nobody told you the objective. The conventional dating rules? They weren't written for your brain.

Profile honesty vs. safety: When do you disclose? There's no perfect answer. Some people put it upfront to filter out incompatible people. Others wait until trust is established. Both have risks. Do what feels safest for you.

First dates and sensory hell: Restaurant dates might be sensory overload. Coffee dates might amp up anxiety. Bars might be too loud. Alternative first dates:

- Walking in a park (movement helps, natural environment, easy escape)

- Activity-based (gives you something to focus on besides social interaction)

- Virtual dates (control your environment)

- Short and specific (one hour at a bookstore)

Communication differences: You might need to explicitly state things neurotypical people hint at. "I like you and want to see you again" instead of hoping they pick up signals. "I need to go home now because I'm overstimulated" instead of making excuses.

Attachment patterns: Your BPD traits might create intense attachments quickly. Your autism might need lots of time to trust. Your ADHD might forget to maintain contact. Understanding your patterns helps you communicate them.

Rejection sensitivity: Dating involves rejection. With RSD, each rejection might feel catastrophic. Build recovery protocols. Have friends on standby. Remember that incompatibility isn't personal failure.

Finding your people: Dating apps for neurodivergent folks exist. Spaces where neurodivergent people gather increase your chances of meeting someone who gets it. But also: neurotypical people who are genuinely accepting exist too.

Long-Term Relationships: The Ongoing Navigation

Being in a long-term relationship while multiply neurodivergent means constant navigation and negotiation. Your needs will change. Your capacity will fluctuate. Your partner (neurodivergent or not) will have their own challenges.

Key strategies for sustainable relationships:

Explicit relationship agreements: Assume nothing. Discuss everything. What does commitment mean? How do you handle conflict? What are deal-breakers? What needs are non-negotiable?

Regular relationship check-ins: Don't wait for problems. Schedule regular times to discuss how things are going, what needs adjustment, what's working.

Parallel togetherness: Being in the same space doing different things counts as quality time. You don't always need to interact to connect.

Sensory negotiations: How do you handle different sensory needs? Who compromises when? How do you create spaces for both/all people's needs?

Communication adaptations: Maybe serious conversations happen better in writing. Maybe you need processing time before responding. Maybe you need explicit confirmation of tone. Find what works.

Support beyond each other: No one person can meet all needs. Friends, family, therapists, communities – multiple support sources protect the relationship from overload.

Parenting When You Can Barely Adult

If you're parenting while multiply neurodivergent, first: you're doing something incredibly hard, and you're probably doing better than you think. Second: your neurodivergence isn't a parenting deficit – it's a different parenting style that can offer unique gifts.

Challenges and solutions:

Executive dysfunction meets child needs: Kids need consistency you struggle to provide. Solutions: Visual schedules for everyone, automated reminders, backup plans, asking for help.

Sensory overload meets sensory children: Kids are sensory intense. Solutions: Sensory breaks built into routine, tag-team parenting when possible, noise-canceling headphones while supervising.

Emotional dysregulation meets child emotions: Kids' emotions might trigger yours. Solutions: Your regulation first (oxygen mask principle), teaching co-regulation, modeling repair after rupture.

Social navigation: School events, playdates, parent social expectations. Solutions: Choose your battles, find your fellow weird parents, advocate for your needs too.

Your neurodivergence might mean your kids grow up knowing:

- Different doesn't mean wrong
- Everyone's brain works differently
- Accommodations are normal
- It's okay to have needs
- Adults aren't perfect

If your kids are also neurodivergent (genetics are strong), you might understand their needs in ways neurotypical parents couldn't. Your struggles become roadmaps for supporting them better.

Finding Your People: Community as Survival

Community isn't optional when you're multiply neurodivergent – it's survival. The isolation of being misunderstood is literally deadly. Finding your people, whether online or in-person, can be lifesaving.

Online communities offer:

- 24/7 availability
- Anonymity if needed

- Specific niche communities (ADHD autistics, neurodivergent BPD, etc.)
- Global perspectives
- Low sensory demands
- Control over interaction level

In-person communities offer:

- Embodied connection
- Local resources
- Immediate support
- Shared activities
- Practice for in-person interaction
- Deeper relationships

Building community might mean:

- Starting where you are (even if that's bed on your phone)
- Finding one safe person and building from there
- Joining groups around special interests
- Attending neurodivergent-specific events
- Creating community where none exists
- Accepting that your community might look different

Navigating Healthcare with Complex Presentations

Healthcare when you're multiply neurodivergent is often traumatic. Providers who don't understand, treatments that don't consider all conditions, communication styles that don't match – it's exhausting. But you need and deserve competent care.

Strategies for better healthcare experiences:

Provider selection:

- Ask explicitly about experience with adult neurodevelopmental conditions
- Look for neurodivergent-affirming providers
- Consider multiple specialists vs. one generalist
- Be willing to switch if it's not working

Communication preparation:

- Write everything down beforehand
- Bring someone for support/advocacy if possible
- Ask for written summaries after appointments
- Record appointments if allowed
- Use patient portals for written communication

Advocacy strategies:

- "I need you to consider how my autism/ADHD/BPD affects this"
- "Standard treatment hasn't worked because of my neurodivergence"
- "I need accommodations to access care"
- "My presentation might not be typical because..."

Managing medical trauma:

- Acknowledge that medical trauma is real
- Build in recovery time after appointments
- Have support people on standby
- Create medical crisis plans

- Know your rights

Building Support Networks That Actually Support

Not all support is supportive. Well-meaning people might offer help that makes things worse. Building effective support networks means being specific about what actually helps.

Effective support might look like:

- Body doubling without talking
- Parallel processing of problems
- Practical help without judgment
- Understanding without fixing
- Presence without demands
- Acceptance of your fluctuating capacity

Building your network:

- Start with one safe person
- Be specific about needs
- Offer reciprocal support you CAN provide
- Accept that some people won't get it
- Keep boundaries with unsafe people
- Remember that online support counts

Support network mapping:

- Crisis support (who can help immediately)
- Daily support (regular check-ins, body doubling)
- Professional support (therapists, doctors, coaches)
- Peer support (others with lived experience)

- Practical support (help with tasks)

- Joy support (people who share your interests)

Communication Scripts for Hard Conversations

Sometimes you need actual scripts because finding words in the moment is impossible. Here are templates to adapt:

Disclosing to friends/family: "I want to share something important about how my brain works. I'm autistic/ADHD/have BPD traits. This means [specific impacts]. I'm telling you because [reason]. What I need from you is [specific support]."

Setting boundaries: "I care about our relationship AND I need [specific boundary]. This isn't about you – it's about my neurological needs. Can we work together to find a solution?"

Asking for accommodations: "I need [specific accommodation] because of my neurodivergent traits. This would help me [specific benefit]. How can we make this work?"

Repair after rupture: "I was dysregulated when [event]. My neurodivergence contributed to [what happened]. I take responsibility for [your part] and would like to repair. Can we talk about how to prevent this?"

The Reality of Neurodivergent Relationships

Here's the truth: relationships while multiply neurodivergent will always require more intentionality, more communication, and more creativity than neurotypical relationships. That's not a flaw – it's just reality. But that intentionality can create deeper understanding, that communication can build stronger connection, and that creativity can lead to relationships that truly fit who you are.

Your relationships might include:

- Periods of distance while you regulate

- Different ways of showing love

- Unconventional relationship structures

- More explicit negotiations

- Different intimacy patterns

- Creative solutions to common problems

The people who matter will work with you to figure it out. The ones who won't? They're telling you they're not your people. Listen to them.

Relationship Needs Inventory

Assess your needs in relationships:

Communication needs:

- Preferred methods (text, voice, in-person)

- Processing time requirements

- Clarity level needed

- Frequency preferences

Physical/sensory needs:

- Touch preferences and boundaries

- Shared space requirements

- Sensory considerations

- Physical intimacy patterns

Emotional needs:

- Reassurance frequency

- Independence vs. togetherness

- Conflict resolution style

- Emotional support type

Practical needs:

- Structure vs. flexibility

- Shared responsibilities

- Financial arrangements

- Future planning

This inventory becomes your relationship roadmap, helping you communicate needs and recognize compatible partners.

Having established these coordinates for building supportive relationships and communities, you're equipped with practical tools for thriving with your unique neurodivergent profile.

Epilogue

Integration and Moving Forward

You've made it through a challenging exploration of three overlapping conditions that affect millions but confuse even experienced clinicians. That alone deserves recognition. Understanding the tangled web of Quiet BPD, ADHD, and autism isn't just an intellectual exercise—it's the foundation for building a life that actually works for your brain.

So where do you go from here?

Your Brain Isn't Broken

Let's start with the most important truth: your complex, beautiful brain doesn't need fixing. It needs understanding.

For years, you've probably heard messages about what's wrong with you. Too sensitive. Too reactive. Can't focus. Can't connect. Too rigid. Too scattered. The contradiction itself felt like evidence of personal failure. How could you be both too much and not enough at the same time?

Now you know. These aren't character flaws or moral failings. They're the predictable results of neurological differences interacting in specific ways. Your brain processes information differently, experiences emotions with different intensity, navigates social situations with different tools, and manages attention through different systems than the statistical average.

Different doesn't mean damaged.

When you have overlapping features of Quiet BPD, ADHD, and autism, your experience naturally contains contradictions. You seek connection intensely while finding social interaction exhausting.

You need routine while struggling to maintain it. You feel emotions deeply while having difficulty identifying them. You mask extensively while desperately wanting to be authentic.

These aren't paradoxes requiring resolution. They're the reality of a nervous system with multiple atypical features operating simultaneously. Understanding this changes everything.

Research consistently shows that self-acceptance—truly accepting your neurological reality without judgment—predicts better outcomes than any specific treatment approach. People who stop fighting their brain's fundamental nature and instead work with it report higher quality of life, stronger relationships, and better mental health across multiple studies.

This doesn't mean giving up on growth or change. It means directing your energy toward accommodations, strategies, and environments that support how your brain actually works rather than trying to force it into a neurotypical mold that will never fit.

The Neurodiversity Paradigm and Your Identity

The neurodiversity movement offers a fundamentally different framework for understanding your experience. Instead of viewing autism, ADHD, and even aspects of BPD through a purely medical or deficit-based lens, neurodiversity recognizes neurological differences as natural human variation.

This perspective doesn't deny that certain features can be disabling or cause genuine suffering. Sensory overload is real. Executive dysfunction is real. Emotional dysregulation is real. These experiences require support, accommodation, and sometimes treatment.

But the neurodiversity paradigm challenges the assumption that difference itself equals disorder. Your brain's wiring creates both challenges and capabilities that exist on a spectrum with the broader population rather than representing categorical pathology.

Many people with ADHD and autism identify positively with these conditions as core parts of who they are. They've built communities, cultures, and identities around shared neurological experiences. The neurodiversity movement advocates for acceptance, accommodation, and celebration of neurological differences rather than cure or elimination.

BPD presents a more complex case. Unlike autism and ADHD, which are neurodevelopmental conditions present from birth, BPD develops through the interaction of biological vulnerability with environmental factors, particularly invalidating or traumatic experiences. Many clinicians view BPD symptoms as potentially reversible with effective treatment rather than permanent features requiring lifelong accommodation.

Yet some people with BPD traits—particularly those with the emotionally sensitive temperament underlying the condition— identify aspects of their emotional intensity, perceptiveness, and passion as valuable parts of themselves they wouldn't want to eliminate even if they could. They distinguish between wanting relief from suffering (abandonment terror, chronic emptiness, self-harm urges) while valuing the depth of feeling and connection their emotional system enables.

Where does this leave you?

Your identity is yours to define. You might identify as autistic, ADHD, both, neither, or something else entirely. You might view your emotional intensity as a feature worth preserving or a symptom to eliminate. You might embrace neurodiversity language or prefer medical terminology. You might see yourself as disabled, different, or both.

What matters is finding frameworks that help you understand your experience, connect with supportive communities, and advocate for what you need. The labels matter less than the self-knowledge and self-acceptance they facilitate.

Research on identity and mental health consistently shows that people who develop coherent narratives about their experiences—stories that make sense of their past struggles and current reality—fare better than those who remain confused about who they are and why life has been so hard. The specific content of that narrative matters less than having one that feels true and allows forward movement.

Some people find liberation in neurodiversity identity. Others prefer to view their struggles as symptoms to overcome. Many hold both perspectives simultaneously, accepting certain features as permanent aspects of their neurology while actively treating others as changeable symptoms.

All of these approaches can work. The key is moving from confusion and self-blame toward understanding and self-compassion, whatever framework facilitates that shift.

Continuing Education and Self-Advocacy

Understanding your brain is a lifelong process, not a destination. Neuroscience advances rapidly. New research on autism, ADHD, and personality constantly refines our understanding. What we know today will be expanded, revised, and sometimes overturned by future discoveries.

Staying informed serves you well. Follow reputable sources that translate research into accessible language. Organizations like the Child Mind Institute, the National Institute of Mental Health, and university research centers regularly publish understandable summaries of new findings. Advocacy organizations for autism and ADHD provide both scientific information and lived experience perspectives.

But continuing education isn't just about consuming research. It's about deepening self-knowledge through ongoing observation of your own patterns, needs, triggers, and capacities.

What helps your nervous system regulate? What throws it into chaos? What environments support your best functioning? What relationships nourish versus drain you? What accommodations make daily life manageable? What situations require masking versus allowing authenticity?

These answers evolve over time. What worked at 25 might not work at 35. Life stages, stress levels, relationship status, work demands, and countless other factors shift the equation. Continuing education includes learning from your own experience across the lifespan.

Self-advocacy builds directly from this knowledge. Once you understand what you need, you can ask for it—from partners, family members, friends, employers, healthcare providers, and social services systems.

Effective self-advocacy requires several skills:

Knowing your rights. Laws like the Americans with Disabilities Act, the Individuals with Disabilities Education Act, and various employment regulations provide protections and accommodations for people with autism, ADHD, and sometimes mental health conditions. Understanding what you're legally entitled to strengthens advocacy efforts.

Communicating clearly. Translate your internal experience into language others can understand. Instead of "I can't handle this," try "The fluorescent lighting creates sensory overload that makes concentration impossible. Can we meet in a different room or allow me to wear sunglasses?" Specific requests get better responses than general distress.

Knowing when to disclose. You're not obligated to share diagnostic information with everyone. Strategic disclosure—sharing with people who need to know and can help—protects both your privacy and your access to support. Some situations require disclosure for legal protections; others benefit from keeping information private.

Building support networks. Self-advocacy doesn't mean doing everything alone. Connecting with others who share similar neurological profiles provides emotional support, practical strategies, and collective advocacy power. Online communities, local support groups, and social media spaces offer various ways to find your people.

Accepting imperfect systems. Healthcare, education, and employment systems weren't designed with neurodivergent people in mind. You'll encounter ignorance, bias, and barriers. Some advocacy efforts succeed; others fail despite your best efforts. This isn't personal failure—it's structural ableism requiring collective action to change. Do what you can while recognizing system limitations aren't your fault or responsibility to fix alone.

The goal isn't fighting every battle or changing every mind. It's creating enough understanding and accommodation in your immediate environment to support your wellbeing and functioning.

A Message of Hope Grounded in Research

Here's what the research actually shows about outcomes:

For BPD: Longitudinal studies following people with BPD diagnoses over decades consistently demonstrate significant improvement over time. Approximately 85% of people diagnosed with BPD achieve remission of symptoms within 10 years. After remission, relapse is rare—only about 10% of people who achieve remission later meet diagnostic criteria again.

This improvement happens both with and without specific BPD treatment, though evidence-based therapies like DBT and MBT accelerate the process and reduce suffering during the journey. The natural trajectory bends toward improvement as people age, develop better coping skills, and create more supportive life circumstances.

The chronic emptiness, abandonment terror, and identity confusion that define BPD in young adulthood typically soften substantially by midlife. The emotional storms calm. The desperate relationship patterns settle. The self-harm urges fade. This isn't wishful thinking—it's robust empirical finding replicated across multiple countries and research teams.

For ADHD: While ADHD is a lifelong neurodevelopmental condition, outcomes vary tremendously based on access to proper diagnosis, treatment, accommodations, and support. When people with ADHD receive appropriate medication, learn effective strategies, and create supportive environments, they achieve success across all life domains at rates approaching the general population.

The key word is "appropriate." ADHD requires individualized, multimodal treatment combining medication (if helpful), behavioral strategies, environmental modifications, and often therapy to address secondary issues like anxiety or low self-esteem. When all these pieces align, people with ADHD thrive in careers, relationships, and creative pursuits.

Recent research increasingly emphasizes ADHD strengths—creativity, ability to hyperfocus on engaging tasks, crisis management skills, out-of-the-box thinking, and entrepreneurial success. These aren't consolation prizes for having ADHD but genuine capabilities the ADHD brain enables.

For Autism: Outcomes research in autism has historically been limited by methodological problems, but recent studies painting a more nuanced picture show that autistic people can and do lead fulfilling, successful lives when provided appropriate support and accommodation rather than forced normalization.

The autism rights movement challenges outcome measures focused solely on appearing neurotypical (eye contact, elimination of stimming, social conformity) in favor of metrics actually related to wellbeing—self-acceptance, autonomy, meaningful relationships, access to accommodations, freedom from abuse, and quality of life as defined by autistic people themselves.

Research shows that late-diagnosed autistic adults, despite often facing significant challenges from years without understanding or support, report relief and improved mental health following diagnosis. Understanding brings clarity, self-compassion, connection to community, and ability to advocate for accommodations that actually help rather than continuing to struggle alone.

Importantly, research on autistic people who've learned to "mask" or "camouflage" their autism reveals this adaptation comes at significant cost to mental health. The pressure to appear neurotypical correlates strongly with anxiety, depression, burnout, and suicidality. Conversely, environments allowing authentic autistic expression without forcing conformity to neurotypical norms support better outcomes.

For overlapping presentations: When features of autism, ADHD, and BPD co-occur, outcomes depend heavily on accurate recognition and appropriate, integrated treatment. The research here is newer and less extensive, but emerging findings suggest that people who receive comprehensive assessment identifying all relevant features fare better than those misdiagnosed or partially diagnosed.

Understanding the full picture allows targeted treatment addressing each contributing factor while recognizing how they interact. DBT skills help manage BPD features. ADHD medication and strategies address executive dysfunction. Autism accommodations reduce daily stress. Together, these approaches create the foundation for substantial improvement.

The message here isn't that everything will be easy or that all struggles disappear. It's that improvement is genuinely possible, expected, and supported by scientific evidence—not just inspirational stories or positive thinking.

You're not facing a life sentence of unchanging suffering. With proper understanding, support, treatment, and time, most people with these conditions see significant positive change. The path forward exists and has been walked successfully by many others before you.

My Integration Story

I spent years convinced something was fundamentally wrong with me in ways I couldn't articulate or fix. The harder I tried to be "normal," the more exhausted and despairing I became. Relationships felt simultaneously essential and impossible. Work required constant masking that left me depleted. Sensory experiences others barely noticed sent my nervous system into overdrive.

Getting accurate diagnoses—first ADHD, then autism, finally recognizing BPD features—didn't magically solve everything. But it shifted everything. Suddenly my experience made sense. The contradictions had explanations. The struggles weren't moral failures but predictable results of how my brain processes the world.

Treatment helped. Medication for ADHD improved executive function enough to maintain basic life organization. DBT skills provided tools for managing emotional intensity without self-destruction. Autism accommodations reduced daily stress from sensory and social demands. Therapy helped process trauma and build healthier relationship patterns.

But honestly? The biggest change came from self-acceptance. Stopping the constant war against my own neurology freed up enormous energy for actually building a life that works for my brain rather than against it.

I still struggle. Sensory overload still happens. Executive dysfunction still derails plans. Emotional intensity still overwhelms. But now I understand why, have strategies that help, and most importantly, no longer interpret these experiences as evidence of personal inadequacy.

I've built a life with enough structure to prevent chaos but enough flexibility to prevent claustrophobia. Work accommodates my needs. Relationships understand my communication style. Environment supports sensory regulation. It's not perfect—perfection isn't the goal—but it's sustainable in ways life never was before understanding my brain.

The relief of finally making sense to yourself cannot be overstated. That's what I hope this book offers you: the clarity to understand your experience, the knowledge to seek appropriate help, and the self-compassion to stop fighting who you fundamentally are.

Moving Forward

You're standing at a choice point. Behind you lies confusion, self-blame, and strategies that never quite worked because they addressed the wrong problems. Ahead lies a path of understanding, appropriate treatment, accommodation, and self-acceptance.

The journey forward requires several commitments:

Commitment to accurate understanding. Keep learning about your brain. Seek competent assessment if you haven't already. Challenge diagnoses that don't fit your experience. Pursue comprehensive evaluation recognizing complexity.

Commitment to appropriate treatment. Find providers who understand overlapping presentations. Try evidence-based approaches long enough to assess effectiveness. Make treatment decisions informed by research rather than convenience or assumptions.

Commitment to self-compassion. Treat yourself with the kindness you'd offer a friend facing similar challenges. Recognize that struggle isn't weakness. Understand that needing support isn't failure.

Commitment to authenticity. Reduce masking where safe. Build environments and relationships allowing genuine self-expression. Connect with communities embracing neurodiversity.

Commitment to advocacy. Ask for accommodations you need. Educate people in your life about your reality. Participate in collective efforts making systems more accessible.

Commitment to patience. Change takes time. Recovery isn't linear. Some days will feel like going backward. Trust the process while taking necessary action.

Your brain is complex. Your experience is valid. Your struggles are real. Your capacity for growth is genuine. The path forward exists and has been successfully walked by many others with similar neurology.

The goal isn't becoming someone else. It's becoming fully, authentically yourself—understood, supported, and accepted in all your neurodivergent complexity.

That journey begins now, with the knowledge you've gained and the self-awareness you've developed. The rest unfolds one day, one choice, one moment of self-compassion at a time.

Your life doesn't have to remain a confusing puzzle. The pieces fit together once you understand the picture they're creating. That picture might look different than you expected, might not match standard templates, might require explaining to others who don't immediately understand.

But it's your picture. Your brain. Your life. Your path forward.

Walk it with confidence, grounded in understanding, supported by evidence, and guided by self-acceptance. The future you're building starts here.

What You Now Know

You understand the overlapping presentations of Quiet BPD, ADHD, and autism—how they interact, where they diverge, why they're so often confused, and what makes your experience unique.

You recognize the importance of comprehensive assessment that looks beyond surface symptoms to underlying mechanisms, considers developmental history, and acknowledges complexity rather than forcing simple diagnostic categories.

You know what evidence-based treatment looks like for each condition and how to integrate approaches addressing multiple features simultaneously rather than treating conditions in isolation.

You have frameworks for understanding yourself that replace confusion and self-blame with clarity and self-compassion, recognizing your struggles as neurological reality rather than personal failing.

You can advocate for yourself armed with language to describe your experience, knowledge of appropriate accommodations, and understanding of your rights within various systems.

You're connected to hope grounded in research showing that outcomes genuinely improve with proper understanding, support, and time—not just inspirational stories but empirical evidence.

This knowledge changes everything. Not because it eliminates challenges but because it transforms your relationship to them. You're no longer fighting in the dark against invisible enemies. You understand the territory, have tools for navigation, and know the destination is reachable.

The rest is practice, patience, and persistence. Keep going

References

1. American Psychiatric Association. (2022). Diagnostic and statistical manual of mental disorders (5th ed., text rev.).

2. Baker, A. E., Lane, A., Angley, M. T., & Young, R. L. (2008). The relationship between sensory processing patterns and behavioral responsiveness in autistic disorder: A pilot study. Journal of Autism and Developmental Disorders, 38(5), 867–875.

3. Barkley, R. A. (2020). Taking charge of adult ADHD (2nd ed.). Guilford Press.

4. Ben-Sasson, A., Hen, L., Fluss, R., Cermak, S. A., Engel-Yeger, B., & Gal, E. (2009). A meta-analysis of sensory modulation symptoms in individuals with autism spectrum disorders. Journal of Autism and Developmental Disorders, 39(1), 1–11.

5. Bunford, N., Evans, S. W., & Langberg, J. M. (2018). Emotion dysregulation is associated with social impairment among young adolescents with ADHD. Journal of Attention Disorders, 22(1), 66–82.

6. Cassidy, S., Bradley, L., Shaw, R., & Baron-Cohen, S. (2018). Risk markers for suicidality in autistic adults. Molecular Autism, 9, 42.

7. Chapman, L., Rose, K., Hull, L., & Mandy, W. (2022). "I want to be like everyone else": Understanding the needs and experiences of neurodivergent adults in intimate relationships. Autism, 26(3), 765–777.

8. Chapman, R., & Botha, M. (2023). Neurodivergence-informed therapy. Developmental Medicine & Child Neurology, 65(3), 310–317.

9. Crowell, S. E., Beauchaine, T. P., & Linehan, M. M. (2009). A biosocial developmental model of borderline personality: Elaborating and extending Linehan's theory. Psychological Bulletin, 135(3), 495–510.

10. Fassbinder, E., Schweiger, U., Martius, D., Brand-de Wilde, O., & Arntz, A. (2016). Emotion regulation in schema therapy and dialectical behavior therapy. Frontiers in Psychology, 7, 1373.

11. Fleming, S. M., Weil, R. S., Nagy, Z., Dolan, R. J., & Rees, G. (2010). Relating introspective accuracy to individual differences in brain structure. Science, 329(5998), 1541–1543.

12. Gaigg, S. B., Cornell, A. S., & Bird, G. (2018). The psychophysiological mechanisms of alexithymia in autism spectrum disorder. Autism, 22(2), 227–231.

13. Gates, J. A., Kang, E., & Lerner, M. D. (2017). Efficacy of group social skills interventions for youth with autism spectrum disorder: A systematic review and meta-analysis. Clinical Psychology Review, 52, 164–181.

14. Gross, J. J. (2015). Emotion regulation: Current status and future prospects. Psychological Inquiry, 26(1), 1–26.

15. Gunderson, J. G., Stout, R. L., McGlashan, T. H., Shea, M. T., Morey, L. C., Grilo, C. M., Zanarini, M. C., Yen, S., Markowitz, J. C., Sanislow, C., Ansell, E., Pinto, A., & Skodol, A. E. (2011). Ten-year course of borderline personality disorder: Psychopathology and function from the Collaborative Longitudinal Personality Disorders study. Archives of General Psychiatry, 68(8), 827–837.

16. Hofmann, S. G., Sawyer, A. T., Witt, A. A., & Oh, D. (2010). The effect of mindfulness-based therapy on anxiety and depression: A meta-analytic review. Journal of Consulting and Clinical Psychology, 78(2), 169–183.

17. Hull, L., Petrides, K. V., Allison, C., Smith, P., Baron-Cohen, S., Lai, M. C., & Mandy, W. (2017). "Putting on my best normal": Social camouflaging in adults with autism spectrum conditions. Journal of Autism and Developmental Disorders, 47(8), 2519–2534.

18. Keenan, E. G., Gotham, K., & Lerner, M. D. (2018). Hooked on a feeling: Repetitive cognition and internalizing symptomatology in relation to autism spectrum symptomatology. Autism, 22(7), 814–824.

19. Kooij, J. J. S., Bijlenga, D., Salerno, L., Jaeschke, R., Bitter, I., Balázs, J., Thome, J., Dom, G., Kasper, S., Nunes Filipe, C., Stes, S., Mohr, P., Leppämäki, S., Casas, M., Bobes, J., McCarthy, J. M., Richarte, V., Kjems Philipsen, A., Pehlivanidis, A., … & Asherson, P. (2019). Updated European Consensus Statement on diagnosis and treatment of adult ADHD. European Psychiatry, 56(1), 14–34.

20. Lai, M. C., Kassee, C., Besney, R., Bonato, S., Hull, L., Mandy, W., Szatmari, P., & Ameis, S. H. (2019). Prevalence of co-occurring mental health diagnoses in the autism population: A systematic review and meta-analysis. The Lancet Psychiatry, 6(10), 819–829.

21. Linehan, M. M. (2014). DBT Skills Training Manual (2nd ed.). Guilford Press.

22. Miller, I. T., Wiederhold, B. K., Miller, C. S., & Wiederhold, M. D. (2020). Virtual reality air travel training with children on the autism spectrum: A preliminary report. Cyberpsychology, Behavior, and Social Networking, 23(1), 10–15.

23. Robertson, A. E., & Simmons, D. R. (2013). The relationship between sensory sensitivity and autistic traits in the general population. Journal of Autism and Developmental Disorders, 43(4), 775–784.

24. Sedgewick, F., Hill, V., Yates, R., Pickering, L., & Pellicano, E. (2016). Gender differences in the social motivation and friendship experiences of autistic and non-autistic adolescents. Journal of Autism and Developmental Disorders, 46(4), 1297–1306.

25. Walker, N. (2021). Neuroqueer heresies: Notes on the neurodiversity paradigm, autistic empowerment, and postnormal possibilities. Autonomous Press.

26. Zanarini, M. C., Frankenburg, F. R., Reich, D. B., & Fitzmaurice, G. (2012). Attainment and stability of sustained symptomatic remission and recovery among patients with borderline personality disorder and axis II comparison subjects: A 16-year prospective follow-up study. American Journal of Psychiatry, 169(5), 476–483.

www.ingramcontent.com/pod-product-compliance
Lightning Source LLC
Chambersburg PA
CBHW051729090426
42738CB00010B/2159